W9-CQC-293

Schizophrenia

CRITICAL ISSUES IN PSYCHIATRY
An Educational Series for Residents and Clinicians

Series Editor: **Sherwyn M. Woods, M.D., Ph.D.**
University of Southern California School of Medicine
Los Angeles, California

A RESIDENT'S GUIDE TO PSYCHIATRIC EDUCATION
Edited by Michael G. G. Thompson, M.D.

STATES OF MIND: Analysis of Change in Psychotherapy
Mardi J. Horowitz, M.D.

**DRUG AND ALCOHOL ABUSE: A Clinical Guide to
Diagnosis and Treatment**
Marc A. Schuckit, M.D.

**THE INTERFACE BETWEEN THE PSYCHODYNAMIC AND
BEHAVIORAL THERAPIES**
Edited by Judd Marmor, M.D., and Sherwyn M. Woods, M.D., Ph.D.

**LAW IN THE PRACTICE OF PSYCHIATRY
A Handbook for Clinicians**
Seymour L. Halleck, M.D.

NEUROPSYCHIATRIC FEATURES OF MEDICAL DISORDERS
James W. Jefferson, M.D., and John R. Marshall, M.D.

**ADULT DEVELOPMENT
A New Dimension in Psychodynamic Theory and Practice**
Calvin A. Colarusso, M.D., and Robert A. Nemiroff, M.D.

SCHIZOPHRENIA
John S. Strauss, M.D., and William T. Carpenter, Jr., M.D.

A Continuation Order Plan is available for this series. A continuation order will bring
delivery of each new volume immediately upon publication. Volumes are billed only upon
actual shipment. For further information please contact the publisher.

Schizophrenia

John S. Strauss, M.D.
Yale University School of Medicine
New Haven, Connecticut

and

William T. Carpenter, Jr., M.D.
Maryland Psychiatric Research Center
University of Maryland School of Medicine
Baltimore, Maryland

Plenum Medical Book Company • New York and London

Library of Congress Cataloging in Publication Data

Strauss, John S.
  Schizophrenia.

  (Critical issues in psychiatry)
  Bibliography: p.
  Includes index.
  1. Schizophrenia. I. Carpenter, William T. II. Title. III. Series.
RC514.S825   616.89′82   81-7321
ISBN 0-306-40704-3   AACR2

To our families

Foreword

When I first read this manuscript, I exclaimed to a colleague: "This is the most important and clinically relevant book on schizophrenia since Bleuler!" Time has not altered my initial enthusiastic evaluation. Drs. Strauss and Carpenter are among the most distinguished researchers in the field of schizophrenia, but they are also clinicians of great experience, breadth, sensitivity, and flexibility. It is from this expertise, as well as their wide familiarity with the world of literature, that they have been able to distill the essence of an exceedingly practical and comprehensive approach to the understanding, evaluation, diagnosis, and treatment of schizophrenia.

They begin by unequivocally stating the inadequacy and futility of approaching schizophrenia via a single model. Standing alone, neither a biomedical, a social, nor a psychological model can adequately account for the complexities of this illness with regard to etiology, phenomenology, course, or optimum treatment. While the advent of psychopharmacological intervention has made a profound impact on both individual treatment and the responsive support systems, and is an important aspect of most treatment plans, to view schizophrenia as a phenothiazine deficiency disease is not only bad science but bad therapeutics.

Their conceptualization of an "interactive developmental systems model" provides a framework upon which to build a broad medical approach to schizophrenia. This model relates variables drawn from different systems, interactive with one another, and contributing to a pathogenetic process across time. Within this bio-social-psychological matrix, one can then organize information relative to vulnerability, the manifest illness *per se*, the course of the disorder, and the multiplicity of factors relative to treatment planning.

Their discussions of diagnostic systems, varieties of schizophrenia and relative prognosis, and the need for a rational and pluralistic approach to the problems of the individual patient are reflective of their own enormous research contributions in these areas, as well as their ability to evaluate fairly and critically the theories and hypotheses of other workers in the field. There is a brilliant critical review of contemporary biological, psychological, and social theories of etiology, a virtual road map through the complexities of evaluating such research in order to separate mythology from probable or proven fact. Neither nihilistic nor unrealistic, they are optimistic with regard to the possibilities of synthesizing a scientific and yet practical clinical approach to these patients. Their approach is always thoughtfully comprehensive and, whether they are addressing the use of drugs or psychotherapy, demands that the clinician's intervention be based on an understanding of the individual patient as opposed to a reflexive response to preconceived notions or theoretical constructs.

SHERWYN M. WOODS, M.D., PH.D.

Preface

Several years ago we agreed to write a book on schizophrenia, believing that some compilation of our published papers laced with editorializing would suffice. We were wrong; the effort to use our vantage as clinician-scientists to translate the body of knowledge on schizophrenia into a readable exposition of value to clinicians, investigators, and clinical administrators proved more challenging than we had anticipated. The process of preparing this book has been rewarding, for it required us to integrate the work of many students of schizophrenia, selecting that information we believed most salient to understanding and treating patients. In that task, we have purposely not prepared an exhaustive treatise or attempted to comment on all relevant work conducted in the field. Rather, we sampled the major findings and examples from a range of clinical and research efforts that have advanced our understanding of the illness.

We have been supported by several institutions and many people during this period, most intimately by our wives, Jane and Carol, and most persistently by our secretaries, Ms. Nancy Ryan and Mrs. Dolores Brocato. A special debt is owed to Dr. Lyman Wynne and Dr. John Romano for their contributions to our development as clinical investigators.

We also wish to express our thanks to Dr. Douglas Heinrichs for his comments on the draft manuscript, to Dr. Ann Pulver and Dr. Howard Zonana for their suggestions on Chapters 6 and 11, and to Dr. Sherwyn Woods and Ms. Hilary Evans for their guidance and patience.

JOHN S. STRAUSS
WILLIAM T. CARPENTER, JR.

Contents

CHAPTER 1

The Concept of Schizophrenia

A clinician is asked to see a young man who is concerned about his restlessness and fears. The young man says that strange noises have been bothering him, and he thinks he knows who is persecuting him. The clinician makes sufficient inquiries to determine that a diagnosis of schizophrenia is warranted, and then—what? Can the diagnosis be confirmed? What does it imply? How should the young man be treated? Will he recover?

Although some speak with certainty and confidence on these issues, these questions have neither obvious nor simple answers. In evaluating such a patient, we can be guided by a particular diagnostic system, and treatment can be based on a particular set of principles. But regardless of how definitive such systems often appear, there comes a time when they must be reevaluated in the light of new information to determine their real validity, error, and incompleteness. For the systems that serve as a basis for dealing with the disorder called *schizophrenia*, this is a time when such a reevaluation is much needed.

Schizophrenic patients with the classical catatonic and hebephrenic syndromes seen by Kraepelin and Bleuler are rarely encountered in many centers treating psychiatric patients; yet, diagnosed schizophrenia continues to be a major cause of anguish and disability. The inevitability of deterioration, supposedly a hallmark of this disorder, has been challenged. Yet, a chronic course with residual symptoms and impaired social functioning is frequently the outcome despite modern treatment. There is increasing information on the importance of genetic, social, family interaction, biochemical, and psychophysiological factors in schizophrenia. But how these variables relate to etiology, course, prevention, and treatment is just being unraveled, and no area of inquiry is so complete at this time as to provide the definitive answer to the puzzle of schizophrenia.

Given the advances in our knowledge and the complexity and incompleteness of the information available, it is important to attempt a synthesis of what is known and to provide a view of schizophrenia that goes beyond a patchwork of isolated Kraepelinian and post-Kraepelinian findings. In this way, as clear a picture as is currently possible can be formed to describe the nature of schizophrenia and its diagnosis, etiology, prognosis, and treatment. Such a reevaluation provides a framework for integrating new information and may also have important implications for improved understanding of other psychoses and even for nonpsychotic psychiatric disorders.

Any attempt at understanding current concepts of schizophrenia must rest on some acquaintance with a historical perspective of this and related disorders. The psychoses generally, and the schizophrenias in particular, were irrevocably set within a medical framework during the nineteenth century and remain there, properly in our view, notwithstanding noteworthy criticisms. During the nineteenth century, physicians were developing disease concepts to replace spiritual and moralistic models to account for behavioral deviance. Especially noteworthy developments occurred in Germany, where the focus was defining specific syndromes. This work centered on the severe psychopathology found in institutional settings, and a large number of seemingly discrete disorders were defined. Of particular relevance to the history of schizophrenia were the illnesses of catatonia, hebephrenia, and paranoia.

Toward the end of the nineteenth century, Emil Kraepelin[1] noted similarities among several of these syndromes, especially their onset during adolescence and young adulthood and a dementia-like end state. He also noted many psychopathological manifestations these disorders had in common, such as disordered thought processes, disruption of the will, and bizarre affect. When Kraepelin conceptually joined hebephrenia, catatonia, and paranoia, calling them *dementia praecox*, he suggested that a common pathological process underlay these various syndromes and provided the basic elements of the concept of schizophrenia used today. The orientation to psychiatric disorder thus established had four key attributes: (a) defining criteria for the disease could be specified; (b) course and outcome could be predicted; (c) a framework for investigating etiology and pathogenesis was provided; and (d) a framework for organizing information on treatment and prevention was established. The introduction of this model has had a profound impact; Kraepelin's discrimination of dementia praecox from manic–depressive illness is a cornerstone of scientific psychiatry.

Eugen Bleuler[2] observed that patients with dementia praecox were not truly demented and suggested that this disorder, which he called "the group of schizophrenias," was characterized by the basic pathological process of splitting in mental associations. Bleuler's contributions included an attempt to specify how this and related psychological processes underlay symptom formation. In doing so, he used psychological processes as well as descriptive features to define the disease, thus broadening the concept to include simple schizophrenia and subsequently a wide range of deviant behaviors. Bleuler and Kraepelin agreed on the major descriptive aspects of the illness, and both believed this to be a disease of somatic origins and poor prognosis.

Since Bleuler's 1911 monograph, the concept of schizophrenia has been widely accepted. Further elaborations of the concept have, in fact, been modest, with relatively minor changes in diagnostic criteria, definition of the syndrome, and specification of subtypes. Major progress in understanding schizophrenia is not reflected in radical alteration of nosology or the concept itself, but rather in the steadily increasing sophistication of methods for research, the findings from these studies regarding the role of biological, psychological, and social variables in schizophrenia, and the development of improved treatment. The most important challenges to the original concept have dealt with prognosis, the classification of brief psychotic reactions, and the original assumption that a single process underlies all forms of the illness—issues that will be discussed in detail in subsequent chapters. Despite the remarkable advances in medical sciences during the twentieth century, however, the underlying etiology and pathogenesis of schizophrenia remain an enigma.

The shift from spiritual and moralistic concepts to medical concepts of the mad was a philosophic step of profound importance. This is not to say that any particular medical model, such as those used by Kraepelin, Bleuler, or many more recent workers in the field, is adequate for synthesizing all information relevant to schizophrenia; nor does it imply that the medical model is universally or uncritically accepted. Some claim that schizophrenia is a myth, and other less extreme critics attribute the deteriorating course to the effects of labeling or societal reaction. Many views of schizophrenia include a social or psychological frame of reference, but these can fit a broad-based medical model, such as the one we will describe in the following chapter. Theories focusing on intrapsychic conflict and on cognitive, learning, social, and cultural paradigms can be situated comfortably within the medical framework, where integration with biological data is facilitated so long as the model is not unduly narrow. These issues are explored at greater length in subsequent chapters.

Although we will discuss "labeling" or societal reaction theories of schizophrenia later in more detail, we should state here our belief that labeling an individual as schizophrenic and the social consequences of many of the behaviors of schizophrenic patients induce reactions and expectations which are antitherapeutic in nature. That is, the course of schizophrenia is complicated by the social reaction to the schizophrenic patient and the assumptions associated with the label. Nonetheless, we also believe that diagnosing schizophrenia serves many useful purposes, such as calling for clinical care rather than legal intervention and providing for communication among scientists and clinicians. We see no convincing evidence that societal reaction theory can account for all psychopathology seen in the schizophrenia syndrome. Further, we think that attempts to dismiss schizophrenia as a myth ignore conspicuous evidence to the contrary.

Since the synthesis of information into a working concept of schizophrenia cannot be accomplished without a point of view, before proceeding to a more detailed discussion of these and other issues in subsequent chapters, it is useful to clarify our bias from the beginning. We believe that schizophrenia is properly viewed in terms of the following principles:

1. Schizophrenia is manifest in individuals as a group of behaviors and mental processes that can be defined with sufficient clarity to provide a reliable and valid distinction between schizophrenia and other established psychiatric syndromes. Some aspects of schizophrenic psychopathology, however, may represent final common pathways and, as such, may overlap extensively with psychopathology seen in other conditions. The presence of schizophrenia does not preclude development of other disorders, nor are schizophrenic patients devoid of ordinary human characteristics—feelings, thoughts, and actions. While some confidence in the functional validity of nosology and diagnostic methods (when carefully applied) is justified, this process is not so precise as to permit uncritical certainty and inflexibility in classification.

2. Schizophrenia is a syndrome comprised of more than one discrete illness. Because of this and because human behavior is complex, there is tremendous variation between individuals in manifest psychopathology and the functional consequences of illness. The boundaries of schizophrenia are not so well defined as the core, and discussion of schizophrenia necessarily includes patients assigned to DSM-III (Diagnostic and Statistical Manual III of the American Psychiatric Association) categories of schizophrenia and schizophreniform psychosis, as well as some patients referred to as having atypical psychoses and schizoaffective psychosis. To facilitate a focused discussion, we exclude any forms of schizophrenia which never result in psychosis, and those very brief psychotic reactions neither preceded nor followed by psychopathological functioning suggestive of schizophrenia.

3. Because social, psychological, and biological processes are involved, it is incumbent upon investigator and clinician to grapple with genetic, biochemical, and neurophysiological mechanisms on the one hand, and psychological, social, and cultural mechanisms on the other. To espouse one while excluding the other is to fail in establishing a sufficiently comprehensive basis for understanding schizophrenia. This is why we insist on a broad medical model as the most suitable framework for conceptualizing schizophrenia. From a practical point of view, no other model is as likely to generate a caretaking and therapeutic stance or to provide a scientific basis for diagnosis and treatment.

4. Patients with schizophrenia vary in their prognostic status, and a full range of outcome functioning is possible. Course of illness is not irrevocably established early in illness, but many factors (often socioenvironmental) interact with the ill individual to facilitate or impede recovery. The clinician has in the treatment armamentarium many interventions which can affect significantly the course of the disease.

In this volume we attempt to provide a framework for the practical integration of information that has accumulated over the years from work with individual patients, from systematic research on schizophrenia, and from other bodies of relevant knowledge. This synthesis may help the clinician, administrator, and investigator to maintain perspective on the complexities involved in the study and care of schizophrenic patients. The following principles serve as guides to some of the issues and views we believe most crucial to understanding schizophrenia. These points will be discussed in detail in the following chapters.

1. The individual with a schizophrenic illness cannot be under-

stood only from the point of view of pathology; personal strengths and environmental circumstances are also extremely important and require specific consideration. Because the patterns of strengths, weaknesses, and circumstances shift over time, assessment of patients must be a continuous process.

2. Clinical observation is the cornerstone of scientific medicine, and the quality of information on which diagnosis, prognosis, understanding, and treatment is based often depends on the quality of the clinical relationship and the clinician's skill as an empathic and informed observer.

3. Treatment goals are multiple and change over time. For this reason, defining a goal only of "treating schizophrenia" is not sufficiently specific. So far as possible, such goals should be specified to enable optimal care and the evaluation of therapeutic success. Multiple therapies are available and may be necessary to meet the multiple goals of treatment. It is unusual for one modality to be selected to the exclusion of others.

4. Since the clinician is faced with the problem of incomplete knowledge regarding etiology and treatment, flexibility and humility are to be valued over rigid guidelines, doctrinaire teaching, and the sometimes excessive intrusions of third-party influences and self-appointed protectors of "patients' rights."

These principles may be self-evident, but it is important to emphasize them because of the frequency with which they are not followed in actual practice. Responses made to explain why the principles are not followed need to be questioned: "We do that already," "That isn't important in this instance," "We don't have the resources." Although these statements may be true to some extent, it has been our strong impression that, even when the principles are accepted in theory, they may be overlooked in practice. This is notable, for example, in reviewing hospital records of schizophrenic patients where no mention is made of social relationship and work problems, in seeing clinics where the continuity of the clinician–patient relationship is not part of the treatment, or in the use of psychotherapeutic modalities without adequate attention to skills training in social relations and work function.

The principles described in this chapter fall short of providing definitive answers to the problems of schizophrenia, but we feel they are more realistic than such answers, given the strengths and limits in available knowledge. An overview of that knowledge and its application to the assessment, treatment, treatment evaluation, and understanding of schizophrenia are presented in the remainder of this volume.

SUMMARY

Since Kraepelin and Bleuler originated the concept of schizophrenia, steady progress has been made in the acquisition of knowledge necessary for understanding this disorder. Despite this progress, the essence of the puzzle remains unsolved. A socio-psycho-biomedical model provides the most suitable framework for conceptualizing schizophrenia, and certain principles can be articulated as guides to the study and care of schizophrenic patients.

RECOMMENDED READING AND REFERENCES

1. Kraepelin, E. *Clinical psychiatry: A textbook for students and physicians,* 7th ed. Translated by A. Ross Diefendorf. New York: Macmillan, 1915.
2. Bleuler, E. *Dementia praecox or the group of schizophrenias.* Translated by J. Zinken (1911). New York: International Universities Press, 1950.

CHAPTER 2

An Interactive Developmental Systems Model of Schizophrenia

Any discussion organizing data relevant to schizophrenia is explicitly or implicitly based on some model or concept of the disorder. Since various concepts have different implications concerning what data are relevant, it is important to describe the concept on which we base our discussion.

We choose a medical model, but one broadly defined. Scientific and sociopolitical factors, as well as our professional backgrounds and experience, dictate this choice. Scientifically, it is our view that the possible alternative nonmedical models do not possess sufficient breadth to incorporate the range of biological, psychological and sociological data relevant to understanding and treating the schizophrenic patient. Regarding social and political considerations, we believe that the aberrant behaviors associated with schizophrenia automatically involve an identification of the patient as deviant and involve a societal reaction to that deviance. This being the case, it is our opinion that a health framework is the orientation most likely to provide a helpful response, a response more benign in its motivation and humane in its assumption of responsibility for the deviant individual than other existing social orientations, such as penal or religious approaches, or neglect. Furthermore, identifying the deviant individual as one suffering from an illness requires a caretaking response which includes acquisition of knowledge relevant to understanding etiology, treatment, and prevention. These enterprises, despite difficulties and shortcomings, have already paid great dividends in providing care for schizophrenic individuals.

Preferring a medical model, we next ask which medical model has the greatest value. A broad model involving social, psychological, and biological factors appears to meet this requirement. Engel has noted that it has become increasingly popular for psychiatrists to affirm their medical background by adhering to a biomedical model of illness, relegating nonorganic aspects of disorder to nonmedical concepts and care systems.[1] This mind/body dichotomization seemed more suitable in past centuries when religion assumed responsibility for the mind and medicine assumed responsibility for the body. Such dualistic thinking ignores the integral relationships between various aspects of human functioning. Nonetheless, some authorities argue that schizophrenia is a neurological disease best treated organically by the neurologist, while interpersonal dysfunction is a problem in living best dealt with by nonmedical psychosocial therapists or educators.

Although specialization can be valuable, dichotomizing schizophrenia along such lines is unfortunate both for clinical practice and research. For the clinician, a biomedical model alone is inadequate to define the problem, to conceptualize diagnosis, treatment, and prevention, or to understand the interacting process involved in mental illness. As an analogy, a biological hypothesis of vascular control may be useful for investigating biological mechanisms involved in a sudden rush of blood to the superficial vasculature of the face, but the clinician would find it wanting as a satisfactory means of incorporating all data relevant to understanding a blush. Similarly, a purely biomedical approach to schizophrenia may have special utility in identifying mechanisms at the biological level involved in vulnerability to illness, symptom formation, or treatment response. However, such an approach will not enable the clinician to understand the origins and meaning of subjective phenomena or deal with those aspects of the disorder manifest as unemployment, anxiety in the context of intimacy, or symptom decompensation in the face of overt hostility.

The biomedical model has proven enormously fruitful in some medical specialties where advances in molecular biology and medical technology are readily applicable, but even here shortcomings of biological exclusivity are being realized.[1] In psychiatry it is difficult to imagine emphasis in one domain (with trivialization, if not denial, of other domains) being optimal, yet models continue to be espoused in which factors from one level of organismic functioning (i.e., biological, psychological, or social) are theorized as central to schizophrenia, essentially ignoring, rather than integrating, other factors. Although the biomedical model is a valuable scientific model of illness, the failure to place biomedical theory and data in an appropriate holistic framework leads to neglect of other areas crucial for understanding mental disorders, generating, for example, a view that understanding the organic basis of brain functioning is sufficient for the medical discipline responsible for the mentally ill. Such a view has undoubtedly contributed to the overuse of drug therapies for schizophrenia today and the overuse of other somatic treatments in the past.

The conceptualization described below assumes that variables from all levels of function are implicated in schizophrenia and requires an integration across levels and across time.

THE INTERACTIVE DEVELOPMENTAL SYSTEMS MODEL OF SCHIZOPHRENIA

An interactive developmental systems model can provide a framework for a socio-psycho-biomedical approach to schizophrenia. This model involves the following:

1. *Interactive* implies causal relationships between variables and sets of variables. The various levels of organization (and factors within each level) interact, and basic processes are altered by these interactions.

2. *Developmental* defines a pathogenic process evolving over time in the context of the individual's childhood, adolescent, and adult development more generally. The interactions between variables noted above are sequential as well as simultaneous. In the earlier phases of the pathogenic process, the issue is vulnerability. Later, manifest illness becomes the focus.

3. *Systems* implies that several sets of independent or semi-independent processes interact to cause schizophrenia and determine its course. Component parts of these systems may be conceptualized as different areas of human function, such as symptoms, social relationships, and work—or as different levels of organization, biological, psychological, and social.

4. *Model* implies a construct for synthesizing information into a coherent whole. Such a model should be useful in specifying relationships between variables, thereby facilitating hypothesis development and testing and refinement of the model's components with eventual verification or disproof of the model itself.

The complexity and heterogeneity of schizophrenia and the amount of missing and incomplete information allow only a sketch of an interactive developmental systems model, but such a sketch will be useful to provide a context for the more detailed information in subsequent chapters. In Figure 1, the model is presented as a logical tree for clarity. The model represents a way of organizing information of relevance to under-

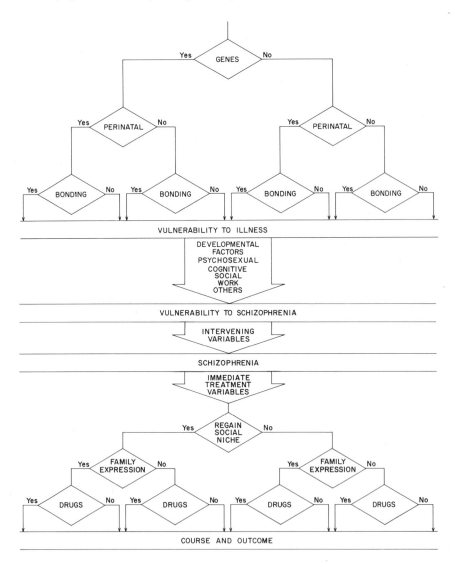

Figure 1. Schema for an interactive developmental systems model of schizophrenia.

standing, for any individual, his relative vulnerability to schizophrenic illness, the development of manifest illness, and the course of disorder.

At the first level is genetic endowment. Investigations have established beyond reasonable doubt that some forms of schizophrenia have a genetic component, although the exact genetic mechanism is unknown, and neither gene nor protein abnormality has yet been defined. The processes that result in the genetically vulnerable person's becoming schizophrenic are also debated, but our model assumes that psychological and socioenvironmental factors interact either to produce or prevent the psychotic state. In those types of schizophrenia such as the acute forms where a genetic component has not been established, we do not assume necessarily that there is no genetic vulnerability. Rather, we suggest that some type of genetically determined attributes may also exist. Some individuals who develop schizophrenia may have no specific genetic vulnerability to the disorder, but in those who do have such vulnerability, it is convenient to suppose that there exist a variety of genetic mechanisms with different degrees of impact.

It goes without saying that many genetically vulnerable individuals will never be afflicted with schizophrenia, or even with any disorders that might be considered as falling within a schizophrenia spectrum. From the moment of conception, the role of environment shapes the future individual, who develops in the context of genetic and environmental interaction. Modification of genetic expression begins inside the protoplasmic environment of the fertilized egg and involves a countless number of intrauterine factors. Which, if any, of these factors bears a causal relationship to schizophrenic vulnerability is not yet determined. But so many factors have an impact on brain development that there will be little reason for surprise if the importance of various mechanisms is established in future investigations.

There is evidence for an association between a variety of perinatal complications and schizophrenia.[2] It cannot yet be determined whether genetic vulnerability is a necessary precondition for perinatal complications to increase vulnerability to schizophrenia, but an interactive developmental concept allows interplay between these vulnerabilities as well as the possibility that each may work independently of the other. An individual not genetically vulnerable may become vulnerable to schizophrenia because of perinatal complications, while another individual may be vulnerable without such complications; and others may have vulnerability from an interaction between genetic and perinatal factors.

In the next schematic step (Figure 1) we identify the initial nurturing relationship. In most societies this bonding relationship is between mother and infant, and the emotional and physical well-being of the offspring is dependent upon successful establishment of this bond.[3] Many factors can impede the optimal development of such a relationship, ranging from the overt catastrophe (e.g., death of the mother) to subtle undermining of the bond, perhaps through unconscious emotional rejection by the mother or defective social responsivity of the infant.

Developmental psychologists and psychoanalysts have described the maturational consequences of various derailments in this bonding process. Many of the postulates that have been generated may be challenged, and further observation is required; but it is evident that this initial social experience has profound implications for the physical and emotional development of the child. It is a reasoned assumption, rather than an established fact, that impediments in the bonding phase of psychological development contribute to vulnerability to schizophrenia.[4] In the individual already vulnerable for genetic, intrauterine, or perinatal reasons, complications here would at least impede the development of the coping mechanisms that might prevent illness or reduce the consequences of illness. It seems more likely, however, that interactions of more specific relevance to the pathogenesis of schizophrenia occur at this stage.

Relying on the body of knowledge contained in developmental psychology and psychoanalysis, particularly Erickson's formulation of maturational task,[5,6] the model depicts psychosexual development as an unfolding process with both simultaneous and sequential interactions within a psychological frame of reference, at the same time springing from an interactive base in ongoing biological development and the social environment.

Information currently being derived from studies of children at increased risk for schizophrenia is beginning to specify these developmental interactions. For example, there is evidence that children vulnerable to subsequent schizophrenic illness may have altered psychophysiological patterns of arousal and reactivity. Furthermore, there is evidence that such vulnerable individuals may manifest deviant neurological and behavioral development. In the model, we represent the cumulative effect of these interacting processes as vulnerability to schizophrenia. We assume vulnerability to be multifactorial with variation from individual to individual, not a precisely definable psychobiological state.

Illness is manifest in some, but not all, individuals vulnerable to schizophrenia. A variety of processes may be conceptualized as interacting with vulnerability to increase or reduce the likelihood of future pathology. The full range of facilitating and preventing factors can be incorporated within this broad medical model. For example, the vulnerable individual may become psychotic when challenged by a natural maturational task or the particular stress of some environmental event. Precipitating events are not only social and psychological but may be biological, such as consumption of amphetamine or even possibly the consequence of a slow virus. In any such circumstances, understanding the precipitating factors requires a synthesizing framework incorporating the various levels of human functioning. For example, knowing the neuropharmacology of amphetamine does not explain how the person became vulnerable to its effects or why he was consuming amphetamine compounds.

Continuing to follow the chronology of the model in Figure 1, we note that course and outcome are not determined merely by the vulnerable individual's developing a schizophrenic psychosis. Once a person is psychotic and the diagnosis of schizophrenia is established, many factors contribute to the course of illness, treatment responsivity, and eventual outcome. The kind of treatment given is one important variable in which the clinician plays a critical role. Other variables include social factors, such as the degree to which society fosters return to health; interpersonal factors, such as the extent to which the familial emotional environment is conducive to health; developmental factors, such as the extent to which preceding functional impairments curtail the patient's capacity to recover; and biological factors, such as the extent to which the relevant brain areas are susceptible to a therapeutic adjustment following pharmacological intervention.

If one does not have an interactive model for schizophrenia, it is difficult for the full range of relevant variables to be considered by the investigator or the clinician. The geneticist knows that multiple factors are involved in determining the eventual consequences of the genetic code, but this fact is ignored by those who assume that a genetically based illness can only be treated somatically. Similarly, genetic data have sometimes been trivialized by those who observe that social and psychological factors play a profound role in schizophrenia.

Failure to use an interactive developmental systems model in the past may have generated unnecessary skepticism and therapeutic rigidity. At the time when patients diagnosed as schizophrenic were presumed to require lifelong custodial care, the social, psychological, and symptomatic outcome was more homogeneous than it is today, when it is assumed that many patients will show symptomatic recovery, that a wide range of functioning outcomes are possible, and that lifelong institutional care is not required. The absence of a complex model may also have encouraged premature conclusions regarding the determinants of schizophrenia. The profound impact of home environment on the course of illness does not argue for a purely psychosocial model of illness any more than the profound impact of anti-psychotic medication on symptomatology argues for a biomedical model.

The interactive developmental systems model represents a way of organizing information relevant to understanding any individual's relative vulnerability to schizophrenic illness, the development of manifest illness *per se,* and the course of the disorder. The model as depicted is incomplete, since no general context for development is given. The interactions within the model do not take place in a vacuum, and some general forces of culture and ecology should be mentioned that provide for the initiation of the processes involved in schizophrenia and the sociobiological matrix in which it unfolds. Such background phenomena as a population's genetic pool, patterns of migration, and assortative mating contribute to understanding the genetic makeup of the individual's biological parents. The familial dynamics of preceding generations, whether the offspring is born to immigrants or natives, socioeconomic status, and other factors provide a backdrop against which human maturation occurs. Of importance also is the nonliving environment which contributes to the biological and psychological development of an individual. Popular examples are nutrition, pollution, and season of birth, with more discrete phenomena, such as infectious disease, incorporated into the model as they specifically apply to an individual. The model itself is illustrated in the figure as though it were a logical tree phenomenon, but this invalid simplification, ignoring possible interactions and feedback loops, is employed only for the sake of clarity.

We trust that the reader of this volume will be left with the impression that while schizophrenia denotes individuals with a disorder involving certain behavioral characteristics, the connotations are as broad and complex as the human experience itself. Despite the fact that schizophrenia remains enigmatic, the broad medical model provides a valuable method for identifying patients and providing help. As a scientific model, it provides an impetus to acquire new knowledge relevant to etiology, pathogenesis, prevention, and treatment. Finally, while discrete medical models such as the biomedical model or psychoanalytic model may have a decisive advantage in guiding specific investigations, a multidimensional model is necessary if the relevance of each discrete point of information is to be put into perspective. Such a model is necessary to the clinician as a guide for considering the full range of information relevant to his role and to the investigator attempting to establish an overview of the processes involved in schizophrenia.

SUMMARY

The various biological, psychological, and social factors in schizophrenia and its treatment require a framework for organizing information and understanding. The interactive developmental systems model emphasizes both the interaction of many factors and the evolution of their impact over time. Although the model is tentative and incomplete, it provides a basis for organizing the complexities involved in schizophrenic disorders.

RECOMMENDED READING AND REFERENCES

1. Engel, G. The need for a new medical model. *Science,* 1975, 196:129–136.
2. McNeil, T. S., and Kaij, L. Obstetric factors in the development of schizophrenia: Complications in the births of schizophrenics and in reproduction by schizophrenic parents. In: *The nature of schizophrenia,* Wynne, L. C., Cromwell, R. L., and Matthysse, S. (eds.). New York: Wiley, 1978, 401–429.
3. Bowlby, J. *Attachment and loss,* Vol. 1. London: Hogarth Press; New York: Basic Books, 1969. Bowlby, J. *Attachment and loss,* Vol. 2. London: Hogarth Press; New York: Basic Books, 1973.
4. Chodoff, P., and Carpenter, W. T., Jr. Psychogenic theories of schizophrenia. In: *Schizophrenia: Biological and psychological perspectives,* Usdin, G. (ed.). New York: Brunner/Mazel, 1975.
5. Erikson, E. *Childhood and society.* New York: Norton, 1963.
6. Erikson, E. Identity and the life cycle. *Psychological Issues,* Monograph 1. New York: International Universities Press, 1959.

CHAPTER 3

Assessment and Diagnosis

The young patient introduced in Chapter 1 has been sitting with an icy stare. The clinician feels uneasy as the stare becomes more hostile. A tense silence is broken by the patient declaring that he will resist all efforts to alter his sex. The clinician asks him to explain, but the patient wonders why the doctor is denying the obvious. Hesitantly at first, the patient proceeds to describe the vague somatic sensations experienced several months ago, sensations which he later realized were caused by drugs in his food. He noticed that his scrotum wrinkled after a cold shower—evidence of an assault on his sexual organs. Sexual thoughts began entering his mind, their source unknown. Last week circumstances converged, fortuitously permitting his sudden discovery of the source of his sexual change. During dinner at his aunt's house, her daughter complained that the food tasted like plastic. His aunt was visibly disturbed but told her daughter that they would discuss it later. Since the aunt had thus unwittingly tipped her hand, it remained only for the patient to account for her motivation. She had always secretly resented the patient's mother and now feared her own daughter's sexual attraction toward the patient. The aunt feared the patient's sexual power, believing he would reunite the family through coitus with her daughter.

The clinician knows the patient is psychotic, but can a specific diagnosis be made? An organic psychosyndrome is ruled out because of the patient's clear sensorium, failure by history to implicate psychoactive drugs, and absence of fever, signs of physical distress, and neurological dysfunction. The clinician observes some dysphoria, but no evidence for mania is noted and the anger, resentment, and anxiety are understandable in the context of an unfolding paranoid psychosis. The presumptive diagnosis is schizophrenia, but how can the clinician be sure?

THE PSYCHIATRIC ASSESSMENT PROCEDURE

Before discussing the decision-making needed for actually reaching the diagnosis, a few points of special importance need to be made regarding the assessment of patients who may be schizophrenic.

1. The focus of the assessment is critical. Early in the evaluation process, the clinician will focus on those features relevant to differential diagnosis and other aspects of psychopathology that are most important for immediate management and treatment decisions. This practical narrowing of attention is guided by the clinician's immediate grasp of the situation and by assumptions concerning what data are relevant to the illness presumed present. With the paranoid young man described above, the clinician will focus initially on information relevant to the differential diagnosis and management of psychotic illness. Determination of the extent to which neurotic anxiety, hypochondriasis, and social apprehension are problems will be postponed.

However, tendencies to maintain such a narrow focus indefinitely, or unjustified assumptions in selecting what information is relevant, can pose major problems. Many attributes important to understanding and treating the patient are ignored by necessity in the urgency of the initial contact, but prolonged disregard of these issues can create serious problems in assessment and treatment. It is our experience that, depending on the bias of the clinician, organic factors, social functioning, family context, and stressful life events are ignored with particular frequency in the assessment of schizophrenic patients.

2. The clinician–patient interaction is central to the diagnostic process. Although the physician may employ a number of ancillary procedures (e.g., neuropsychological testing, EEG, clinical and toxicology evaluation), the foundation of diagnostic assessment is the clinician as participant/observer. It is the information generated in the clinician–patient relationship, rather than any other single source of data, which is decisive in diagnosis and treatment.

3. Security and comfort for clinician *and* patient must be assured to permit the leisure and openness required for quality assessment. While most schizophrenic patients do not become violent, clinicians frequently evaluate patients with the possibility of impulsive behavior in question. When necessary, leaving the office door open or having family or staff join the interview can minimize risk and facilitate information exchange.

As in any clinical interview, using judgment concerning interview style and content and clarifying structure and intent are also important. Failure to take these precautions for ensuring the comfort of clinician and patient can lead to hasty and poorly founded diagnostic and treatment decisions.

4. The initial evaluation should be conceptualized as information exchange rather than as information collection. Some clinicians regard the initial task as an interrogation through which the features of psychopathology required for diagnosis will be exposed. However, the clinician also needs to hear how the patient views his situation and to take this information seriously. Perhaps the patient views his depression as more troublesome than his hallucinations or sees his family context as the most central problem of all. Understanding this view can be crucial to adequate assessment and treatment of the entire problem. During the initial evaluation, as part of the exchange of information, it is also important that the clinician provide information to the patient about the process of assessment and treatment planning.

5. Initial interviewing should provide information on the setting in which illness emerged, and on a range of the patient's strengths and weaknesses in personal and social functioning. This provides a human perspective on illness, something especially important when illness disrupts a sense of self and the patient and those around him react primarily to psychopathology.

6. The clinician should not be so preoccupied or overwhelmed with the patient's anguish, nakedness of impulse, or bizarre thought and behavior that he avoids listening to the full range of the patient's expression, fails to recognize the meaningfulness of the content of psychopathology, does not relate empathically to psychotic experiences, assumes that the patient is incapable of collaborating in assessment, or assumes that the patient is either incapable of or disinterested in receiving information.

CLASSIFICATION AND DIAGNOSTIC CERTAINTY

In discussing diagnosis or any type of classification, reliability and validity are two crucial concepts. Reliability indicates the extent to which different clinicians agree on the diagnosis of a patient. It can be high or low regardless of whether or not a diagnostic category is valid. Although reliability is crucial for clinical communication, good reliability should never be equated with validity, which reflects the extent to which diagnoses define meaningful classes of patients in relation to such criteria as prognosis, etiology, and treatment response. Although a label may sound meaningful on the surface, serious disagreement on how it should be applied or absence of clinical or research validity will give the illusion of communication or knowledge when little or none exists. These concepts of reliability and validity need to be kept in mind in reading the following review of the various diagnostic approaches to schizophrenia and their implications.

Some of the principles used for diagnosing schizophrenia described originally by Kraepelin and Bleuler are presented in Tables 1 and 2. They are, of course, the pioneering statements in the field. Besides their content, however, it will be noted that these are narrative descriptions and thus contrast quite strikingly with the lists of criteria often used in more recently established systems to be discussed below. The narrative form of diagnostic criteria, although clinically more natural, has often caused serious problems for establishing reliability.

Several trends in developing diagnostic criteria have been pursued since the time of Kraepelin and Bleuler. Following Bleuler's emphasis on describing a basic underlying pathological process in schizophrenia, other psychiatrists, especially in the United States, have attempted to classify schizophrenia according to various factors considered common and perhaps basic to the schizophrenic process. For example, it has been suggested that the diagnosis of schizophrenia could be based primarily on the presence of a characteristic thinking disorder, specific "ego" defects, or certain impairments in the capacity for interpersonal relatedness. The previous American Psychiatric Association diagnostic manual, DSM-II, reflects this approach to a considerable extent (Table 3).

The field has recently become disillusioned with such a model as a basis for diagnosing schizophrenia, since no single unifying factor highly discriminating for schizophrenia has been demonstrated definitively. Furthermore, the definitions of attributes, such as the types of thought disorder previously believed to characterize schizophrenia uniquely, have not been sufficiently operationalized to permit their use as reliable diagnostic criteria. The result of these shortcomings is that diagnostic systems based on such supposed underlying characteristics tend to be used in an idiosyncratic fashion.

Table 1
Diagnostic Characteristics of Schizophrenia[a]

"Dementia praecox consists of a series of states, the common characteristic of which is a peculiar destruction of the internal connections of the psychic personality. The effects of this injury predominate in the emotional and volitional spheres of mental life" (p. 3).

"The diagnosis of individual cases of dementia praecox has to distinguish the manifold states from a whole series of diseases which outwardly are similar but which are totally different in their course and issue. Unfortunately, there is in the domain of psychic disorders no single morbid symptom which is thoroughly characteristic of a definite malady. . . . On the other hand, we may expect that the composition of the *entire picture* made up of its various individual features, and especially also the changes which it undergoes in the course of the disease could scarcely be produced in exactly the same way by diseases of a wholly different kind" (p. 257).

Among the symptoms of particular diagnostic importance are catatonic symptoms, especially negativism and mannerisms, "signs of psychic weakness [such as] the want of judgment, the senselessness of the hypochondriacal complaints, the inaccessibility towards the reassuring statement of the physician, the emotional dullness and want of interest, the lack of improvement on relaxation from work, further, the more or less distinct manifestations of automatic obedience or of negativism. Hallucinations and sudden incomprehensible impulsive actions naturally are wholly in favour of dementia praecox" (p. 259).

"Of special importance is the proof that in a certain period of life a change of the whole personality, a deterioration and a failing, has taken place; still, the forerunners of such an 'acquired *folie morale*,' as we have seen, go back even to childhood." (p. 259).

Also diagnostically important are "silly, convulsively unrestrained, or indifferent [moods]" (p. 267).

"The content of the delusions [is important]. The delusion of physical, especially sexual, influence points with great probability, the idea of influence on thought and will almost certainly, to dementia praecox" (pp. 268–269).

The persistence of various peculiarities of behavior during periods of illness that otherwise appear to be remissions are also important diagnostically.

---

[a]Abstracted from E. Kraepelin, *Dementia Praecox and Paraphrenia*. Translated by M. Barclay, from the 8th German edition of the *Textbook of Psychiatry*, Edinburgh: E. S. Livingston, Ltd, 1919.

Table 2
Diagnostic Characteristics of Schizophrenia[a]

"The symptoms must have reached a certain degree of intensity to be of any diagnostic value" (p. 294).

"Characteristic anomalies, indifference, lack of energy, unsociability, stubbornness, moodiness—hypochondriacal complaints, etc., are not necessarily symptoms of an actual mental disease; they are, however, often the only perceptible signs of schizophrenia. It is for this reason that the diagnostic threshold of schizophrenia is higher than that of any other disease; and it is because of this that latent cases are such a common occurrence" (p. 294).

"Only a few isolated psychotic symptoms can be utilized in recognizing the disease, and these, too, have a very high diagnostic threshold value. Manic and depressive moods may occur in all psychoses; flight of ideas, inhibition and—as far as they have not assumed specific characteristics—hallucinations and delusions, are partial phenomena of the most varied diseases" (p. 294).

"Thus the individual symptom in itself is less important than its intensity and extensiveness, and above all, its relation to the psychological setting" (p. 295).

"However, if [certain key symptoms] should appear in a state of full clarity of consciousness, an observer who has carefully evaluated all the circumstances can often establish the diagnosis with certainty from a single such symptom" (p. 295).

"Definite schizophrenic disturbances of association alone are sufficient for the diagnosis" (p. 298).

Severe thought "blocking" and "splitting of personality fragments" are important (p. 298).

"Autism in itself cannot be utilized for the diagnosis" (p. 299).

Other useful, though generally not entirely sufficient, characteristics include "obscurity of concepts," "absence of ability for discussion," "the expression of sudden ideas," "the schizophrenic type of attention" (p. 299). Hallucinations, especially auditory or of bodily sensation, thoughts being heard, delusions of certain content, especially if "poorly thought out, and fragmentary" (p. 300). "The delusion that everyone already knows what the patient is thinking is almost pathognomonic" (p. 300). Also important are "unmotivated affectless laughter" (p. 301) and "stereotypies" (p. 302).

"There are no negative pathognomonic signs that would exclude the existence of schizophrenia" (p. 304).

All these characteristics are described in more detail in several parts of Bleuler's monograph, along with other diagnostic characteristics of value.

---

[a] Abstracted from E. Bleuler, *Dementia praecox or the group of schizophrenias.* Translated by J. Zinken (1911). New York: International Universities Press, 1950.

Table 3
DSM II Diagnostic Description
for Schizophrenia[a]

". . . a group of disorders manifested by characteristic disturbances of thinking, mood and behavior. Disturbances in thinking are marked by alterations of concept formation which may lead to misinterpretations of reality and sometimes to delusions and hallucinations which frequently appear psychologically self-protective. Corollary mood changes include ambivalent, constricted and inappropriate emotional responsiveness and loss of empathy with others. Behavior may be withdrawn, regressive and bizarre. The schizophrenias in which the mental status is attributable primarily to a *thought* disorder are to be distinguished from the Major Affective Illnesses (q.v.) which are dominated by a *mood* disorder. The Paranoid States (q.v.) are distinguished from schizophrenia by the narrowness of their distortions of reality and by the absence of other psychotic symptoms" (p. 33).

[a] American Psychiatric Association, Diagnostic and Statistical Manual II, American Psychiatric Association, Washington, D.C., 1968, used with the permission of the American Psychiatric Association.

SYMPTOM-BASED DIAGNOSES

An alternative approach to diagnosing schizophrenia is to use a few highly discriminating symptom manifestations of the illness as diagnostic criteria. Such a method is not based on theory, but rather on its practical utility in identifying patients with an illness for which laboratory or other objective methods are not available. This approach is found in some German diagnostic schools and in several American centers and has influenced the development of DSM-III.

Kurt Schneider has provided a system most clearly illustrating such a diagnostic approach.[1] In developing this system, Schneider adhered to two basic principles. First, a diagnosis should be based on manifestations of the illness that occur frequently in that illness and rarely in other disorders. Second, diagnostic criteria should reflect manifestations that are readily observable and easily agreed upon by the diagnosing clinicians. Because of these principles, Schneider searched for highly discriminating, frequently occurring, and reliable psychiatric symptoms to serve as a basis for diagnosing schizophrenia.

Schneider's System

Schneider identified eleven symptoms that, except for their occasional presence in organic psychosyndromes, he believed to occur only in

schizophrenia. These symptoms are called "first-rank symptoms" because of their diagnostic importance, not because of any theoretical considerations.

Three of Schneider's eleven first-rank symptoms are special forms of
auditory hallucinations: (1) the patient hears voices speaking his thoughts
aloud; (2) the patient experiences himself as the subject about whom
hallucinatory voices are arguing; and (3) the patient hears hallucinated
voices describing his activity as it takes place. Thus, in contrast to the
practice in many American centers, not all auditory hallucinations are
considered discriminating of schizophrenia.

The fourth symptom, delusional percept, is a two-stage phenomenon consisting of a normal perception followed by a highly personalized
delusional interpretation of that perception. For example, on seeing a salt
shaker, one patient suddenly believed it was a sign that the Pope was
calling him to Rome.

Symptoms 5–11 can be conceptualized as delusions reflecting a deficit
in the barrier separating self from environment. They are as follows: (5)
somatic passivity—the patient is a passive and reluctant recipient of
bodily sensation imposed from the outside; (6) thought withdrawal—the
patient believes that his thoughts are being removed from his mind by an
outside agent; (7) thought broadcast—the patient believes his thoughts
are being magically transmitted to others; and (8) thought insertion—the
patient experiences his thoughts as though they were put into his head by
an external force. The patient described in the opening paragraphs of this
chapter would be diagnosed schizophrenic by Schneider's criteria because he had this symptom. The remaining first-rank symptoms (9, 10,
and 11) consist of affects, impulses, or motor activity experienced as
imposed and controlled from outside one's body.

Although American psychiatrists were generally unfamiliar with
Schneider's concepts until the 1970s, his teachings were accepted as valid
in many centers around the world. His first-rank symptoms of schizophrenia had often been assumed sufficient, or pathognomonic, for diagnosing schizophrenia.

But only recently have empirical investigations of Schneider's first-
rank symptoms been undertaken.[2-6] The weight of the evidence from
these studies, although confirming the reliability of these criteria, does
not support their pathognomonicity. Although all 11 symptoms were
shown to be helpful in discriminating schizophrenia, approximately
10–25% of patients receiving diagnoses of affective disorder, many of

whom had characteristic cyclical patterns of illness with predominant affective components, had at least one first-rank symptom. Patients diagnosed as having paranoia or a paranoid state posed a particular problem, since they frequently had first-rank symptoms, but there is controversy whether these diagnoses should actually be included under the rubric of schizophrenia. These findings were incorporated into the standard diagnostic manual, DSM-III, where first-rank symptoms appear as criteria for schizophrenia and other types of disorder and are not considered as absolutely incompatible with affective illness.

Although the studies cited above demonstrated that, with an approach like Schneider's, reliability in diagnosing schizophrenia can be achieved, the validity of this system appears to be more limited than was originally believed. Besides the findings that these criteria are not usefully viewed as pathognomonic, recent work suggests that the first-rank symptoms have minimal prognostic value.[7,8]

Schneider's diagnostic model deserves particular attention because its clarity, supposedly atheoretical derivation, and wide acceptance form a basis for communication between clinicians of various backgrounds. As a model, it must be distinguished from Kraepelin's approach, which included onset and course data as well as cross-sectional symptomatology in establishing a diagnosis.

Several diagnostic systems have been developed recently to provide operational criteria for the Kraepelinian approach to diagnosing schizophrenia. One of the pioneering efforts is that of Robins and the St. Louis group.[9] The criteria developed by this group are presented in Table 4. This system has given rise to a series of subsequent modifications called the Research Diagnostic Criteria that has been widely used for investigations of schizophrenia.

Another group of recent approaches to defining diagnostic criteria for schizophrenia has viewed this process not so much as working from absolutes, but rather as an empirical bootstrap operation. In establishing the diagnosis of schizophrenia, the key variables of etiological validity, prognosis, and treatment response have been elusive and, as with most mental illnesses, the tools of histopathology, radiology, and biochemistry are not yet useful to confirm a diagnosis. Practically speaking, therefore, establishing diagnostic criteria for schizophrenia can be readily carried out by one of two empirical methods. Theoretically derived diagnostic criteria can be tested for their ability to classify patients who have already been diagnosed according to some accepted, though incompletely

Table 4
Operational Diagnostic Criteria
for Schizophrenia[a]

"Schizophrenia. For a diagnosis of schizophrenia, A through C are required.

"A. Both of the following are necessary: (1) A chronic illness with at least six months of symptoms prior to the index evaluation without return to the premorbid level of psychosocial adjustment. (2) Absence of a period of depressive or manic symptoms sufficient to qualify for affective disorder or probable affective disorder.

"B. The patient must have at least one of the following: (1) Delusions or hallucinations without significant perplexity or disorientation associated with them. (2) Verbal production that makes communication difficult because of a lack of logical or understandable organization. (In the presence of muteness the diagnostic decision must be deferred.)

"(We recognize that many patients with schizophrenia have a characteristic blunted or inappropriate affect; however, when it occurs in mild form, interrater agreement is difficult to achieve. We believe that, on the basis of presently available information, blunted affect occurs rarely or not at all in the absence of B-1 or B-2.)

"C. At least three of the following manifestations must be present for a diagnosis of 'definite' schizophrenia, and two for a diagnosis of 'probable' schizophrenia. (1) Single. (2) Poor premorbid social adjustment or work history. (3) Family history of schizophrenia. (4) Absence of alcoholism or drug abuse within one year of onset of psychosis. (5) Onset of illness prior to age 40."

[a] J. Feighner, E. Robins, S. Guze, R. Woodruff, G. Winokur, and R. Munoz, Diagnostic criteria for use in psychiatric research. *Archives of General Psychiatry*, 1972, 26:57–63. Copyright 1972, American Medical Association.

specified system (e.g. "discharge diagnosis" or "DSM-II diagnosis"). Or one can use a similar group of diagnosed cases but attempt to determine empirically the most effective specific criteria for assigning those patients to the diagnostic groups. The weakness of both methods arises from problems implicit in the "bootstrap" nature of the conception (i.e., in establishing the validity of the initial diagnosis, an issue that will be discussed more fully later in this chapter).

An excellent example of the theoretical–empirical approach to establishing diagnostic criteria is the New Haven Schizophrenia Index. Astrachan and his colleagues,[10] drawing on findings of earlier investigators, constructed a list of symptoms that were expected to be discriminating and were consistent with major theoretical work in the field. This checklist was heavily weighted with items of thought disorder, hallucinations, and delusions but also included ratings of inappropriate affect, paranoid ideas, catatonic behavior, and depersonalization. Using this checklist, a scoring system was designed to differentiate patients who had been diagnosed schizophrenic from those who had not. This procedure resulted in a set of six symptom categories made up of 21 illustrative symptoms, with a specific system for scoring each symptom and category. When this system was applied to several patient groups, Astrachan, et al., had considerable success in correlating high scores on the checklist with a schizophrenic diagnosis and low scores with a nonschizophrenic diagnosis. While this particular system provides a broad definition of schizophrenia, a similar approach, defining schizophrenia narrowly, could just as easily be used.

A FLEXIBLE DIAGNOSTIC SYSTEM

Since the field was already populated with numerous competing systems of diagnosis, we have preferred an empirical approach in our diagnostic research. Using observations made on clinically diagnosed patients, we have employed a broad range of sign and symptom data to determine how best to discriminate between diagnosed schizophrenic and nonschizophrenic patients. We were fortunate to be carrying out these investigations within the International Pilot Study of Schizophrenia (IPSS), since it was a large, multinational study of a kind that has three distinct methodological advantages for this type of research. First, such a study makes available large numbers of patients for hypothesis generating and testing. Second, a systematic data base on patients from diverse cultures is available, lessening the possibility that culture-specific psychopathology or local practices in patient identification will appear as critical variables. If patients from only one center were studied, culture-specific symptom criteria for schizophrenia might result which would be less suitable for diagnosis in other centers.

A third advantage of a large international study is that psychiatrists with divergent backgrounds and biases diagnose patients and describe psychopathology. For this reason, the influence of variables considered as powerful discriminators in one school but trivial in another is reduced. The result is that one can evaluate attributes of schizophrenia that are considered important across diagnostic schools.

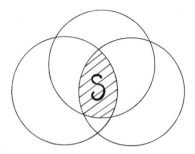

Figure 2. Overlap of diagnostic systems.

The Venn diagram in Figure 2 illustrates these last two points. The shaded area in the center can represent similarities among schizophrenic patients brought together from diverse cultural and socioeconomic backgrounds. Thus, the features of schizophrenia that are more closely related to incidental or local variables will appear outside the shaded area. The same is true when this diagram is considered as illustrating a study design involving psychiatrists from several diagnostic schools. The shaded area would represent those signs and symptoms commonly believed indicative of schizophrenia. For example, if loose associations were considered diagnostic of schizophrenia in one country but not in others, while passivity delusions were regarded as critical indicators of schizophrenia in all countries, then only the latter would fall within the shaded area.

Following this rationale, each of 1,119 IPSS patients was assigned to a schizophrenic or nonschizophrenic category, according to the diagnosis given by the investigators in each center. Of the original 1,202 patients in the study, 83 had been given diagnoses of paranoid state, unspecified reactive psychosis, or paraphrenia and were excluded from analysis, since we had little confidence in assigning these patients to either the schizophrenic or nonschizophrenic group. A country-by-country randomization of patients was carried out to establish a split sample, each half containing approximately 405 diagnosed schizophrenics and 155 diagnosed nonschizophrenics. One half (Group B) was omitted from the initial data analysis (hypothesis-generating), so that it could later be used to replicate or disconfirm (hypothesis-testing) the value of highly discriminating signs and symptoms derived from Group A.

A series of analyses was undertaken with Group A. The sign and symptom data obtained from a standard interview (the Present State Examination) consisted of 230 symptoms and 130 signs which were ar-

Table 5
Flexible System for Diagnosing Schizophrenia

1. Restricted affect	8. Widespread delusions in many areas of patient's life
2. Poor insight	
3. Hearing one's thoughts aloud	9. Incoherent speech
4. Early awakening (−)	10. Unreliable information
5. Poor rapport	11. Bizarre delusions
6. Depressed facies (−)	12. Nihilistic delusions
7. Elation (−)	

rayed for purposes of analysis as 443 overlapping variables. The 443 variables contained numerous single items (e.g., thought broadcast) considered relevant to the distinction between schizophrenia and non-schizophrenia or regarded as having general psychopathological importance (e.g., anxiety). Psychopathological dimensions were also formed by combining related items. Thus, we could analyze a dimension that contained maximum information regarding the presence or absence of depression as well as examine some individual depression items (e.g., depressed facies) for their discriminating power. Analysis of variance and discriminant function analysis were carried out and resulted in the identification of a number of highly discriminating signs and symptoms of schizophrenia.[11]

A number of symptom groups were tested for differentiating schizophrenics from nonschizophrenics,[12] but the most effective was comprised of a group of 12 symptoms (Table 5). To use these, the 9 signs and symptoms more prevalent in schizophrenia are scored one point each if present, and the 3 symptoms—waking early, depressed facies, and elation—more prevalent in the nonschizophrenic group are scored one point each when absent. Thus, the most stringent criteria for our assignment to a schizophrenic diagnosis would be a total score of 12 (i.e., 9

Table 6
Discriminating Power of the Flexible System

Number of symptoms	Percentage patients diagnosed	
	Schizophrenic	Nonschizophrenic
4 or more	91	28
5 or more	80	13
6 or more	66	4
7 or more	44	1

schizophrenic symptoms present and 3 nonschizophrenic symptoms absent).

Table 6 demonstrates that a meaningful split between schizophrenic and nonschizophrenic diagnostic assignments results when one determines that five or more, or six or more, of these symptoms are present. At these levels, a very substantial number of diagnosed schizophrenic patients would be judged schizophrenic, while relatively few of the patients assigned nonschizophrenic diagnoses would be placed in the schizophrenic groups.

The percentages in the left-hand column can guide the clinician on the implications of different levels of stringency in this system for designating a schizophrenic population. For example, 80% of acute and subacute schizophrenic patients might be expected to have at least five of these symptoms. In the right-hand column, the percentages indicate the degree of "error" one might anticipate when making diagnostic assignments solely with the system. For example, if a patient with five or more of these symptoms is assigned automatically to a schizophrenic category, one might expect that 13% of the patients assigned to schizophrenic groups would not be diagnosed as schizophrenic in many centers. Hence, the degree of discordance between clinical diagnosis and system diagnosis provides a built-in estimate of false positive and false negative assignments, thus discouraging any inappropriate application of the system as an absolute indicator of schizophrenia.

Embedding the 12-point system within the framework of a clinical assessment considering all data relevant to diagnosis (e.g., past history, family history, drug response profile) can further reduce false positive assignments. A lithium-responsive patient with a past history of manic and depressive episodes would not be assigned a diagnosis of schizophrenia simply because six points were scored. Thus, the bootstrapping principle indicates that the final integrity of diagnosis depends on the combination of a fully informed clinician rigorously trained in differential diagnosis, employing empirically supported operational diagnostic criteria as much as possible to enhance reliability and validity and to facilitate communication.

The advantages of using the flexible system of diagnosis described above are as follows:

1. The 12 signs and symptoms are operationally defined, and reliable judgments regarding their presence or absence can be made.

2. Cutoff level can be selected according to the particular tasks of the

person using the system. If the goal is to bring some standardization into a busy clinic or emergency room, a point total of 5 might be selected as a level of stringency that is compatible with the need to diagnose most cases. Similarly, a level of 7 points could be used by a research group that is trying to draw 10 "certain" cases from a pool of 50 patients already diagnosed as schizophrenic. Here the goal is to eliminate erroneous assignments to schizophrenia rather than to diagnose all or most cases.

3. The system is simple enough to encourage its use by various clinical and research groups in describing their subjects, thus enhancing the opportunity for comparability of groups in clinical communication and in replication studies.

4. Since this system is intended to supplement rather than replace ordinary clinical diagnosis, increased reliability may be obtained without an untoward reduction in the clinical basis for diagnosis. Discordant cases (i.e., where system and clinical diagnosis disagree) are flagged for special attention rather than merely reassigned from one class to another. This approach explicitly differs from "diagnosis by criteria" or "Chinese menu" approaches associated with some diagnostic systems.

Like other sets of specified diagnostic criteria, this 12-point system has the potential to increase reliability and reduce misunderstanding in clinical communications. Even so, we cannot expect a completely homogeneous patient group to emerge, regardless of how stringent the symptom criteria are that are chosen. As suggested by the model described in Chapter 2, schizophrenia as defined by symptom criteria is almost certainly not a single illness with uniformity of cause or course. For example, even when one of the several approaches to subtyping schizophrenia is used, with only one exception efforts have not produced a high degree of course and outcome homogeneity. That exception involves utilizing either duration of illness or premorbid characteristics as diagnostic criteria. Such an addition has many ramifications that may not be immediately obvious. Some of these will be discussed below, and the premorbid adjustment subtypes specifically will be discussed in Chapter 5.

BEYOND A SYMPTOM-BASED DIAGNOSIS

Notwithstanding the values of the diagnostic system described above, there are a number of theoretical and practical limitations to any diagnosis of schizophrenia based on symptom criteria alone. Empirically, it has been found that symptoms of schizophrenia do not define a homogeneous population in terms of genetics, function, outcome, or indications for treatment. From a practical viewpoint, this means that the clinical value of diagnoses based exclusively on symptom criteria is limited. Theoretically, symptoms alone rarely constitute an adequate basis for defining a disease; the concept of disease implies an underlying pathological process with ramifications far beyond symptom description.

For these reasons, our field requires a more comprehensive approach to diagnosing schizophrenia than is provided by cross-sectional symptom methods such as those described above. The disease entity approach, as used by Kraepelin, is one solution. This approach subsumes etiology, course of illness, outcome, and signs and symptoms data within diagnosis. Such an approach is well suited when a single illness is defined with extensive similarity on these various dimensions across patients. It has serious limitations currently in considering schizophrenia, since a single illness is not defined; etiology is not known; and pattern, manifest psychopathology, and outcome vary so much among patients.

The multiaxial approach to diagnosis[13] is an alternative to the disease entity approach mentioned above. A multiaxial system defines several dimensions relevant to diagnosis, assuming a significant degree of independence among axes. The dimensions or axes other than symptoms can include such characteristics as duration of illness, social relations function, work function, and precipitating events (see Table 7). Each patient is described in terms of all axes, each axis providing distinct information of

Table 7
A Multiaxial System for Diagnosis[a]

Axes
  1. Symptoms
  2. Course of disorder
  3. Associated life events
  4. Social relations function
  5. Work function

[a] J. Strauss, A comprehensive approach to psychiatric diagnosis, *American Journal of Psychiatry*, 1975, 132(11):1193–1197.

relevance to clinical assessment. Optimally, data from all axes would jointly define diagnosis.

There are several advantages to such a system. Empirically, it appears that the various axes may in fact be independent, so that no single label can be even descriptively accurate. Prognostically, symptom type, social relations function, work function, and prior duration of illness have all been demonstrated as having independent predictive value. And in terms of treatment, each axis has many of its own implications regarding patient problems and strengths important for treatment planning. Besides these advantages, multiaxial diagnosis, with its several biological, psychological, and social dimensions, provides a natural, operational basis for a biopsychosocial orientation and for dealing with multiple etiologies and treatment methods. If, as seems likely in schizophrenia, several causative factors operate simultaneously or more than one treatment needs to be used at the same time, the multiaxial approach provides a structure for thinking and acting in the multivariable context required.

A modified multiaxial approach has been used in DSM-III. This diagnostic system defines five axes: (1) syndrome, (2) personality disorder, (3) associated physical illness, (4) psychosocial stressors, and (5) level of adaptive function in the past year. These axes are somewhat different from those depicted in Table 6, reflecting the fact that several multiaxial systems have been suggested, and no one set of axes has yet been demonstrated to be definitively more valid or useful than others.

The modification in DSM-III from a pure multiaxial format is that preeminence is given to one of the axes, axis 1 syndromes. Given the current orientation in psychiatry, it is probably necessary, as a first step, to assign a patient to a diagnostic class based predominantly on symptoms and signs. Assessing a patient on the other dimensions may play a secondary role in bringing more information into classification. This modification in DSM-III arises from the fact that, despite their etiological, prognostic, and treatment validity, the dimensions, other than signs and symptoms, have a somewhat uncertain role in terms of traditional classification. For example, prior duration of illness is of vital importance prognostically and for treatment planning, but it does not indicate *what* illness is present. Tobacco addiction and schizophrenia cannot be differentiated by chronicity data alone.

This two-step multiaxial approach in which one axis is preeminent permits two options. The axis carrying the primary diagnostic data may be "pure" (i.e., sign and symptom data only), keeping course, social functioning, or etiological data independent in other axes. Or, the first step may involve data from various axes such as symptoms, poor social functioning, and chronicity, combining in the first axis to classify a patient as schizophrenic. This conforms to a disease entity approach supplemented by further recording of data on semi-independent dimensions. It is this latter option which is used in the DSM-III classification of schizophrenia (Table 8). This provides maximum data for step one but has the disadvantage of assuming that such a disease entity is valid and renders the other axes no longer independent. DSM-III schizophrenia cannot be validated by chronic course and social dysfunction, for these factors (a minimum limit on duration of disorder and social impairment) are now part of the definition of schizophrenia.

Their recent development notwithstanding, multiaxial systems, perhaps better than any other approach, emphasize the point that, while signs and symptoms provide the most readily applicable diagnostic data, clinical assessment must include more information about the individual patient before a proper appreciation of the psychopathology can be obtained. The chapters on prognosis and treatment discuss these issues further.

SUBTYPES OF SCHIZOPHRENIA

The history and heterogeneity of the "group of schizophrenias" has encouraged efforts to define subtypes. Three disorders, hebephrenia, catatonia, and paranoia, previously designated as separate disorders, were brought together by Kraepelin in constructing the concept of *dementia praecox*. These disorders continue as the preeminent subtypes, but many alternatives and modifications have been suggested and occasionally adopted. Of these, many have been around the boundary lines of the "core" schizophrenic syndrome. Of this peripheral group, the most vexing is simple schizophrenia, the most confusing are latent and pseudoneurotic schizophrenia, the most dissatisfying is residual schizophrenia, and the most heuristically important is schizoaffective schizophrenia.

Other attempts focusing on the boundary line of schizophrenia have been made to distinguish nonschizophrenic functional acute psychoses from schizophrenia; the most notable efforts in this area since Kraepelin's fundamental differential of manic–depressive insanity being Langfeldt's

Table 8
DSM III Criteria for Schizophrenia[a]

Diagnostic criteria for a schizophrenic disorder:

A. At least one of the following during a phase of the illness:

1. Bizarre delusions (content is patently absurd and has no possible basis in fact), such as delusions of being controlled, thought broadcasting, thought insertion, or thought withdrawal.

2. Somatic, grandiose, religious, nihilistic, or other delusions without persecutory or jealous content.

3. Delusions with persecutory or jealous content if accompanied by hallucinations of any type.

4. Auditory hallucinations in which either a voice keeps up a running commentary on the individual's behavior or thoughts or two or more voices converse with each other.

5. Auditory hallucinations on several occasions with content of more than one or two words having no apparent relation to depression or elation.

6. Incoherence, marked loosening of associations, markedly illogical thinking, or marked poverty of content of speech if associated with at least one of the following:

    a. Blunted, flat, or inappropriate affect.

    b. Delusions or hallucinations.

    c. Catatonic or other grossly disorganized behavior.

B. Deterioration from a previous level of functioning in such areas as work, social relations, and self-care.

C. Duration: continuous signs of the illness for at least six months at some time during the person's life, with some signs of the illness at present. The six-month period must include an active phase during which there were symptoms from A, with or without a prodromal or residual phase.

D. The full depressive or manic syndrome (criteria A and B of major depressive or manic episode), if present, developed after any psychotic symptoms or was brief in duration relative to the duration of the psychotic symptoms in A.

E. Onset of prodromal or active phase of the illness before age 45.

F. Not due to any organic mental disorder or mental retardation.

[a]Abstracted from Diagnostic and Statistical Manual III, American Psychiatric Association, Washington, D.C., 1980, and used with the permission of the American Psychiatric Association.

schizophreniform psychosis,[14,15] cycloid psychosis,[16] the acute reactive psychoses of Scandinavia,[17] and the episodic dyscontrol psychoses.[18] Metabolic, toxic, and drug-induced psychoses are not considered under functional psychoses, but some such syndromes have been discerned among presumed schizophrenic patients; amphetamine psychoses, anticholinergic crises, and psychedelic-induced psychoses are present-day examples.

In our view, it is necessary to deal with simple, latent, and pseudoneurotic subtypes by requiring the presence of psychotic symptoms suggesting schizophrenia at some point of illness and hence considering these conditions as outside the realm of schizophrenia. This does not deny the possibility of a subpsychotic or even subclinical schizophrenia, but we cannot presently identify such cases reliably.

It has been possible to test the generally recognized subtypes, paranoid, catatonic, hebephrenic, acute, simple, and schizoaffective, for descriptive validity.[19] Work reported in Volume 1 of the IPSS[4] had already suggested that various subtypes were similar rather than distinct in their psychopathological manifestations. Using different methods with the same data base, consisting of relatively acute and subacute patients, we determined that paranoid, hebephrenic, acute, and schizoaffective subtypes were essentially similar in signs and symptoms when depicted across 27 psychopathological dimensions. Catatonics had more bizarre and disordered behavior, and simple schizophrenics were quite low in psychosis ratings. These results called into question the general usefulness of applying subtype designations, at least for relatively acute and subacute schizophrenic patients. It is possible that descriptive distinctions are only valid in the chronic stages, and Leonhard and Kleist have contributed elaborate subclassification schemes for chronic schizophrenia.[20] On the other hand, workers such as Schneider simply speak of schizophrenia without reference to subtype.

We believe the traditional subtypes are of limited usefulness and validity. Not only are distinctions among living patients less pronounced than textbook descriptions, but patients simultaneously manifest the psychopathology of several subtypes and/or change from one subtype to another in subsequent episodes of illness. Although traditional subtype distinctions have seemed at times to have promising associations to genetic, biochemical, psychophysiological, or treatment response data, such relationships are neither clear nor strong and usually do not stand up to replication. An exception appears to be the schizoaffective subgroup.[21] But it is not yet clear how much the course of illness, drug response, and family history of illness findings in studies of this subtype are accounted for by an acute/chronic distinction combined with diagnostic approaches which overdiagnose schizophrenia, thereby including cases of affective illness which are then subtyped as schizoaffective.

Welner's report, for example, finds a similar course of illness between "chronic" schizophrenic patients and "chronic" schizoaffective patients.[22]

The most important subdivision now possible in schizophrenia distinguishes between patients with good and poor prognoses. Prior duration of illness contributes to this distinction once sufficient time elapses following onset, but an emphasis on premorbid social functioning seems even more valid. Poor premorbid patients have a worse prognosis and may have more biological abnormalities and different treatment needs from good premorbid patients. In fact, some believe that good premorbid patients with their relatively good prognosis may not even have "true" schizophrenia. In any case, the premorbid adjustment dichotomy (or continuum) appears to be an extremely important one and needs to be considered routinely by the clinician and the investigator, even though it is not a central part of standard diagnostic manuals. The prognostic implications of premorbid adjustment are further discussed in Chapter 5.

Biological subtyping of schizophrenic patients is now being attempted by many investigators, and clinicians may soon have ancillary data from the genetic biochemistry laboratory (e.g., monoamine oxidase activity), the psychophysiology laboratory (e.g., evoked potential), or the nuclear medicine/radiology laboratory (e.g., CAT scan) relevant to etiological or treatment subgroups.

DSM-III continues the use of the traditional, although renamed and redefined, subtypes in schizophrenia. Of more profound significance in DSM-III is the fact that schizophrenia is defined as a chronic or subchronic illness, and the more acute psychoses labeled "schizophrenia" in DSM-II are now in a class titled "Psychoses Not Elsewhere Classified," with the following major types: (1) schizophreniform psychosis, (2) schizoaffective psychosis, (3) brief reactive psychosis, and (4) atypical psychosis.

The cross-sectional symptom criteria used in DSM-III for defining schizophrenia are also used to define DSM-III schizophreniform psychosis. This contrasts with Langfeldt's original concept of schizophreniform psychosis, which he believed could be differentiated by the distinctive characteristic symptoms found only in schizophrenia. In fact, DSM-III uses similar diagnostic symptoms for schizophrenia and all four of the "Psychoses Not Elsewhere Classified" listed above.

Is the patient described in this volume really schizophrenic? We have tried to show in this chapter how much that decision must depend on what diagnostic criteria are chosen. In one study,[23] it has been shown that from a sample of 272 first-admission psychiatric patients, anywhere from 68 to 4 patients might be considered as schizophrenic, depending on the criteria used. There is less divergence with more chronic patients, where concordance between diagnostic systems is greater.[24,25]

There is certainly no reason for total despair. Many studies have now demonstrated that reliable diagnostic criteria for schizophrenia can be defined. The International Pilot Study of Schizophrenia has demonstrated that schizophrenia can even be reliably identified across many centers and that there is at least some consensus about a core group of such patients and the associated diagnostic criteria. In fact, through the efforts of many clinicians and investigators, diagnostic progress is now marked by the existence of improved descriptive diagnostic systems for schizophrenia, such as that in DSM-III. These provide a valuable basis for using the concept and assessing the relative validity of different diagnostic approaches. On the other hand, absolutism in the diagnosis of schizophrenia has such a shaky base as to cast doubt about the critical capacities of any unflinching proponent. It is more prudent to accept the advantages of systems such as DSM-III without presuming validity beyond that demonstrated.

A final cautionary note: Clearly specified criteria for diagnosis may discourage in-depth training in psychopathology. The clinician's experience, inquiry into, and intuitive grasp of the nature of psychopathology can incorporate a full range of relevant information. Criteria should guide, discipline, and challenge, but not curtail, the clinical diagnostician.

SUMMARY

Progress in the classification of schizophrenia is a bootstrap affair, requiring the development of reliable criteria and the testing of these criteria against measures of their etiological, descriptive, prognostic, and treatment validity. The task is complicated further by the way in which approaches to evaluating patients can screen in or out whole areas of information that may be potentially important.

In spite of these problems, sets of clear diagnostic criteria have been formulated and are being evaluated. Furthermore, there tends to be considerable agreement about a core group of patients who would be considered schizophrenic, as shown by the flexible diagnostic system. Multiaxial diagnoses provide a system for combining such symptom-based criteria with a wide range of other important characteristics. The new standard diagnostic manual of the American Psychiatric Association—DSM-III—combines clear criteria and a multiaxial diagnostic framework reflecting the current advances in this still developing area.

RECOMMENDED READING

Bleuler, E. *Dementia praecox or the group of schizophrenias.* Translated by J. Zinkin. New York: International Universities Press, 1950.

Carpenter, W. T., Jr., and Strauss, J. S. Cross-cultural evaluation of Schneider's first-rank symptoms of schizophrenia. *American Journal of Psychiatry,* 1974, 131(6):682–687.

Goffman, E. *Asylums.* New York: Anchor Books, 1961.

Jaspers, K. *General psychopathology.* Translated by J. Hoenig and W. Hamilton. Manchester: Manchester University Press, 1963.

Kraepelin, E. *Dementia praecox.* Translated by R. M. Barclay. Edinburgh: ES Livingston Ltd., 1919.

Schneider, K. *Clinical psychopathology.* Translated by M. W. Hamilton. New York: Grune & Stratton, 1959.

Strauss, J. S. A comprehensive approach to psychiatric diagnosis. *American Journal of Psychiatry,* 1975, 132(11):1193–1197.

World Health Organization. *The international pilot study of schizophrenia,* Vol. 1. Geneva: WHO Press, 1973.

REFERENCES

1. Schneider, K. *Clinical psychopathology.* Translated by M. W. Hamilton. New York: Grune & Stratton, 1959.
2. Mellor, C. S. First-rank symptoms of schizophrenia. *British Journal of Psychiatry,* 1970, 117:15–23.
3. Carpenter, W. T., Jr., Strauss, J. S., and Muleh, S. Are there pathognomonic symptoms of schizophrenia? *Archives of General Psychiatry,* 1973, 28:847–852.
4. World Health Organization. *The international pilot study of schizophrenia,* Vol. 1. Geneva: WHO Press, 1973.
5. Carpenter, W. T., Jr., and Strauss, J. S. Diagnostic issues in schizophrenia. In: *Disorders of the schizophrenic syndrome,* L. Bellak (ed.). New York: Grune & Stratton, 1980.
6. Koehler, K. C. The diagnosis of schizophrenia. Part 2: Reliability and validity of modern research criteria. *Weekly Psychiatry Update Series,* Lesson 12, 1979.

7. Hawk, A. B., Carpenter, W. T., Jr., and Strauss, J. S. Diagnostic criteria and five-year outcome in schizophrenia. *Archives of General Psychiatry*, 1975, 32:343–347.

8. Kendell, R. E., Brockington, I. F., and Leff, J. P. Prognostic implications of six alternative definitions of schizophrenia. *Archives of General Psychiatry*, 1979, 36:25–31.

9. Feighner, J., Robins, E., Guze, S., Woodruff, R., Winokur, G., and Munoz, R. Diagnostic criteria for use in psychiatric research. *Archives of General Psychiatry*, 1972, 26:57–63.

10. Astrachan, B. M., Harrow, M., Adler, D., *et al.* A checklist for the diagnosis of schizophrenia. *British Journal of Psychiatry*, 1972, 121:529.

11. Carpenter, W. T., Jr., Strauss, J. S., and Bartko, J. J. Flexible system for the diagnosis of schizophrenia. *Science*, 1973, 182:1275–1278.

12. Carpenter, W. T., Jr., Strauss, J. S., and Bartko, J. J. Use of signs and symptoms for the identification of schizophrenic patients. *Schizophrenia Bulletin*, Winter, 1974:37–49.

13. Strauss, J. S. A comprehensive approach to psychiatric diagnosis. *American Journal of Psychiatry*, 1974, 132(11):1193–1197.

14. Langfeldt, G. *The prognosis in schizophrenia and the factors influencing the course of the disease.* Copenhagen: E. Munksgaard, 1939.

15. Langfeldt, G. Schizophrenia, diagnosis and prognosis. *Behavioral Science*, 1969, 14:173–182.

16. Perris, C. A study of cycloid psychosis. *Acta Psychiatrica Scandinavica*, Supplement 253, 1974.

17. Mitsuda, H. (ed.). *Clinical genetics in psychiatry: Problems in nosological classification.* Tokyo: Igaku Shoin, 1967.

18. Monroe, R. R. *Episodic behavioral disorders: A psychodynamic and neurophysiologic analysis.* Cambridge: Harvard University Press, 1970.

19. Carpenter, W. T., Jr., Bartko, J. J., Carpenter, C. L., and Strauss, J. S. Another view of schizophrenia subtypes. *Archives of General Psychiatry*, 1976, 33:508–516.

20. Fish, F. J. *Schizophrenia.* Bristol: John Wright & Sons, Ltd., 1962.

21. Pope, H., and Lipinski, J. Diagnosis in schizophrenia and manic–depressive illness. *Archives of General Psychiatry*, 1978, 35:811–828.

22. Welner, A., Croughan, J., Fishman, R., and Robins, E. The group of schizoaffective and related psychoses: A follow-up study. *Comprehensive Psychiatry*, 1977, 18:327–332.

23. Strauss, J. S., and Gift, T. E. Choosing an approach for diagnosing schizophrenia. *Archives of General Psychiatry*, 1977, 34:1248–1253.

24. Overall, J. E., and Hollister, L. E. Comparative evaluation of research diagnostic criteria for schizophrenia. *Archives of General Psychiatry*, 1979, 36:1198–1205.

25. Stephens, J. H., Ota, K. Y., Carpenter, W. T., Jr., and Shaffer, J. W. Diagnostic criteria for schizophrenia: Prognostic implications and diagnostic overlap. *Psychiatry Research*, 1980, 2:1–12.

CHAPTER 4

Beyond Diagnostic Criteria

THE PATIENT'S EXPERIENCE OF SCHIZOPHRENIA

In the previous chapter, we focused on considerations of patient assessment particularly important for diagnosis. A medical framework emphasizes diagnostic and prognostic implications of the patient's symptoms, signs, and other clinical characteristics; but beyond these basic considerations, a broad range of the patient's experiences of schizophrenia require careful attention. Detailed interest in these experiences may reward the concerned clinician or investigator with important clues to the nature of schizophrenia and to factors central in pathogenesis and recovery.

As in so many issues relating to schizophrenia, the field is polarized regarding intensive exploration of patient experiences and the utility of such data in providing useful clues to the nature of basic pathological processes. For example, in regard to possible underlying meanings of delusional material, Jaspers,[1] apparently remote from intensive clinical contact with patients, argued that schizophrenic experiences could not be understood because the empathic bond necessary for one person to perceive another's experience was absent. Symptoms were viewed as useful markers of pathological processes, but not as a source of direct or detailed information about underlying meaning. Freud,[2] although his experience with schizophrenic patients was also limited, considered that such persons could not be investigated psychoanalytically because they were unable to establish a transference relationship. This view, like that of Jaspers, has discouraged two generations of clinicians and investigators from intensive explorations of the experiences of persons with schizophrenia.

Thus, many have considered the inner experiences and views of schizophrenic patients as incomprehensible and of limited value for understanding the processes involved in the disorder. This view is often unwittingly demonstrated in case conferences, for example, when no inquiry is even made into the patient's impressions of the sequence or sources of symptoms or their relationship to personal circumstances. It is as though the disorder were not a human condition connected with life situations and their meaning for the individual. The other extreme of this polarity is represented by clinicians and theorists who find that intensive exploration of schizophrenic experience does reveal meaningful connections between symptom content and intrapsychic conflict and believe that causal mechanisms in schizophrenia are thus demonstrated.

This polarization in regard to schizophrenic experiences appears to reflect a Cartesian dichotomizing of mind and brain. Such a dichotomy denies the intricate relationship between biological and psychosocial processes. We believe that studying the views and experiences of patients is a cornerstone of clinical inquiry relevant to both domains. Detailing the processes of subjective experience offers a wealth of data relevant to the biology, psychology, and sociology of the illness. With present knowledge, these data are particularly valuable for the important task of hypothesis development, but they will rarely provide information adequate for definitive proof.

In this chapter, we shall focus on only three areas of detailed experiential information, areas that are often neglected but may hold important keys for treatment and research. These areas are: the patient's feelings about the schizophrenic experience, the symbolic implications of symptoms, and the patient's experience of sequences defining onset, exacerbation, treatment impact, and recovery processes.

SUBJECTIVE FEELINGS ABOUT THE SCHIZOPHRENIC EXPERIENCE

Beyond the existence of the symptoms themselves, what does it feel like to have these experiences, to have schizophrenia? Poets, playwrights, novelists, and filmmakers have frequently portrayed the disintegrating fear sometimes described by individuals losing their grasp on reality. However, detailed accounts of such experiences are available only from patients and clinicians who have been willing to explore the depths of psychosis.[3-12]

Before describing some of the most striking aspects of these reports, a brief review of schizophrenic symptoms is necessary in order to set the context for this discussion. The schizophrenic patient is subject to the impact of symptoms affecting all areas of functioning. Cognition may be disturbed by disorganized thinking, intrusive thoughts, or the involuntary withdrawal of thoughts. Other less clearly defined experiences such as muddled, blurred, or increasingly slowed thoughts may also occur. Thought content can be taken over by organized or fragmented delusions of many kinds, or by delusional mood—an eerie sense that things are not quite what they seem, accompanied by a readiness to create delusional interpretations. Strange perceptual experiences include not only hallucinations in one or more sense modality, but other perceptual phenomena to which less attention has often been paid. Among these are the feeling that objects are getting larger or smaller, are receding physically into the distance, have strange colors, or are no longer clearly delineated.

A wide range of affective disturbances can occur.[13] Restricted or flattened affect is a hallmark of process or chronic schizophrenia, and inappropriate or labile affect is frequently noted. But patients who fail to demonstrate emotionality, or who demonstrate it inappropriately, may have powerful and meaningful private feelings. This has been particularly well described by Searles.[7] In fact, depression, sadness, shame, guilt, anxiety, panic, happiness, elation, smugness—in short, the range of human emotion—is part of the experience of schizophrenic persons. The relevance of these various emotions for diagnosis, monitoring the course of illness, and understanding schizophrenia is again being recognized.[10,13,14]

Besides symptoms in all modalities, important combinations of disturbances occur. For example, affective/cognitive interaction is distorted or diminished in many patients, confusing the meanings and altering the significance of everyday life. Any person reading, conversing, or observing is automatically grasping meaning and assessing intent and importance. When cognitive function and emotional responsivity are distorted, the essence of meaning is undermined. It is worth noting that symptoms as experienced by patients may not fall into the neat groupings[15] that some approaches to psychopathology suggest. And patients report intermediate systems that fall, for example, somewhere between thoughts (delusions) and voices (hallucinations) or between hallucinations and normal perceptions.[16]

And what is the person's inner world like that is associated with these symptoms, symptom combinations, and symptom blends?

1. *Perplexity.* Not surprisingly, one of the most common feelings patients report is perplexity, uncertainty as to where voices are coming from, why thoughts are intruding or disappearing, or where control originates that dominates actions and volition.

2. *Isolation.* Another commonly described feeling in subjective reports of schizophrenic patients is the sense of isolation. There appear to be several possible origins of this feeling. In some instances it appears to follow estrangement resulting from feeling so different or inhuman because of the symptoms themselves. McDonald[17] describes the horror of isolation following a psychotic experience and the wonderful feeling of being understood by friends who had used psychotomimetic drugs. In other instances, the feeling of isolation may precede the onset of psychotic symptoms by years, suggesting that its origins were not from the symptoms experienced, but from some more longstanding process.

The estrangement following the occurrence of symptoms of being stigmatized as a "schizophrenic" or psychiatric patient may be particularly powerful and permanent.[18,19] For some patients, the interpersonal void is replenished by the friendliness and companionship of hallucinated voices.[20] Other persons may find social links with patients, treatment personnel, family members, friends, and co-workers.

3. *Terror.* Another very common subjective experience reported is terror. Such a feeling may be generated by the hearing of a hallucinated voice, the feeling that someone else has gained total control over one's mind, one's thoughts, or the entire world, or by practically any of the schizophrenic symptoms.

But these are only brief descriptions of individual feelings, and no such description can do justice to the richness and pathos of these experiences. For this reason, we strongly advise the reader to consult at least one of the suggested autobiographical accounts of schizophrenia listed at the end of this chapter.

What implications do these kinds of experiences have? To begin with, it is crucial for the assessment process that the clinician acquire a sense of the impact of schizophrenia on the patient's subjective life. Because of the individuality of the experiences, only careful attention by listening, inquiry, and empathy can provide this data. It is important, for example, that the clinician be aware if the patient is experiencing the stark terror that can occur when a person feels he is losing his mind. Differentiating this state from the anxiety and smugness that may accompany a patient's conviction that powerful forces are being unleashed by his thoughts is important in determining the steps necessary for treatment.

Second, the clinician's ability as a participant–observer to perceive such emotions serves as foundation for the clinical relationship. The initial view of the patient's subjective status may be misleading, and the task of "feeling one's way into the shoes of another" is an ongoing process. For example, a patient's initial belligerence may serve to enforce a social distance, leaving others unaware of the loneliness and despair that are felt.

Third, the clinician's interest in, and awareness of, the patient's subjective experiences also can reduce the patient's sense of isolation and provide a basis for helping the family, treatment staff, and others to understand and deal with their own misconceptions and distancing.

Finally, the patient's feelings about his experiences may provide important clues to the nature of psychological, social, and biological processes involved, clues that are crucial to the clinician and the investigator. Issues such as biologically and/or psychologically determined problems in managing high stimulus levels or response tendencies to difficult social situations can be highlighted by attempting to understand the patient's subjective experience.

POSSIBLE SYMBOLIC IMPLICATIONS OF SYMPTOMS

Are the symptoms of schizophrenia symbolic reflections of basic feelings and conflicts in the patient's life? Might a delusion of being influenced by mysterious forces, for example, be the expression of conflict about an intrusive parent?

As we noted earlier, it is crucial to prevent the issue of possible symptom meaning from degenerating into a choice between psychosocial and biological determinants of schizophrenia. No total allegiance to psychodynamic etiological theory is required to assert that content and timing of symptoms in schizophrenia are potentially informative regarding issues of psychosocial development, stress, and conflict. The issue is not that these aspects of disorder necessarily determine the occurrence and form of illness, but that content of illness experiences can be explored to help the patient make as much sense of the experiences as possible. Psychotic patients have difficulty gaining a realistic perspective, and "sorting things out" from a personal reference point can reduce the sense of alienation and incompetence. Inquiring into the possible meaning sources of a particular symptom may help the patient understand his perplexing experiences and the stresses that precipitate them. The treatment implications of the possible symbolic meanings of symptoms will be discussed further in Chapter 9.

PATIENTS' VIEWS OF SEQUENCES DEFINING ONSET, EXACERBATION, TREATMENT, AND RECOVERY PROCESSES

Detailed patient reports of the sequences of their experiences provide potentially valuable information about a wide range of issues. These issues include pathogenesis, personal vulnerabilities and strengths, and environmental factors that may be of major clinical and research importance.

Sequences in Onset and Exacerbation

In describing the beginnings of disorder, patients often provide considerable information about the evolution of their symptoms.[21] Changes of intensity and constancy in stimuli are sometimes noted just before the onset of delusions and hallucinations. For example, some patients experience an increased volume of sounds prior to onset of auditory hallucinations; other patients become less able to ignore peripheral stimuli or tangential ideas just before the onset of disordered thought. These experiences suggest that fragmentation of basic perceptual, attentional, and ideational functions may be precursors to the more commonly noted symptoms of schizophrenia. Such fragmenting of mental functioning—recalling Bleuler's fundamental symptoms of dissociative thinking—may reflect early stages in a single progressing pathological process.

Another sequential aspect of patients' experience around the onset of schizophrenia may also suggest cause–effect relationships in pathological processes. In the account by Sechehaye,[3] the patient's vague feelings of unreality and lack of control over her environment appeared to evolve into full-blown delusions of being controlled by some outside force. On occasion, these delusional ideas then appeared to become "more real" by becoming voices, as though auditory hallucinations in some instances might be delusions that had become more severe.

A patient reported to us that, as isolation and distance from others increased, she felt less and less a part of the real world. Increasing isolation merged into derealization and depersonalization, and she began to experience delusions of passivity. When she felt she was losing contact with the real world (and thus was not in control of her environment), she observed that things continued to happen. Therefore, she reasoned, someone else must be in control, directing events and her own thoughts and actions. This delusion of passivity, pathognomonic for schizophrenia according to Schneider and "incomprehensible" according to Jaspers, perhaps can be placed in an understandable perspective through attention to the sequence of events. These experiences are very similar to those described by Sartre[22] and, in a very different context, by Freeman and Melges[23] in their study of disintegration in the sense of time.

Attention to the detailed sequence of patient experiences around onset may also give clues to psychobiological developmental factors in the occurrence of schizophrenia. A schizophrenic boy in his late teens described lifelong detachment from his peers and other people around him, a report confirmed by his family. During his teens, however, he began to wish for more involvement. As he sought for and developed relationships, he became more involved and felt more alive. But this appeared to increase ideational, affective, and perceptual stimulation and was soon followed by fragmentation of perception and ideation, which in turn was succeeded by delusions and hallucinations.

Careful temporal dissecting of such experiences provides a basis for generating hypotheses about the interplay of biological, psychological, and social factors in pathogenesis. One could suggest that the early isolation this adolescent boy described protected him from overwhelming stimulation—stimulation at levels that might have been disorganizing, perhaps suggesting impaired psychosocial and/or neurophysiological modulating mechanisms. The lifelong history suggests that the basic defect was innate or occurred early in development, preceding by years the symptomatic expression of schizophrenia. This brief example simply sketches the potential basis for hypothesis generation and theory building from such reports. Of course, speculations can be endless, but clear delineation of the patient's experiences can provide the most trustworthy foundation for generating such conceptions. From these, it is possible to move—while keeping in touch with clinical data—toward more fully developed hypotheses and hypothesis testing.

TREATMENT AND RECOVERY

Patients' descriptions of event sequence may also provide major clues to the processes of treatment impact and recovery. For example, in the *Autobiography of a Schizophrenic Girl*, [3] Renee's descriptions of phasing into and out of reality may be instructive regarding the kinds of treatment and other environmental factors that either assist patients in returning to reality or push them away from it. The state of the relationship between patient and therapist seemed in this instance to be significantly associated with the type and severity of symptoms. When the therapist got too close or was too kind, the delusions of outside control quickly intensified. At the opposite extreme, the therapist's absence was often accompanied by Renee's believing that the world was totally empty. In noting another interpersonal aspect of treatment, Jefferson[4] describes the important motivating force of the doctors and the nurses who almost challenged her to be sane. In fact, many accounts suggest that increased motivation to get well, often stimulated by an interpersonal experience, is vitally involved in the recovery process.[17,18]

Detailed reports by patients of the sequences in their experiences may reflect stages in the recovery process. Are there such stages? Are these similar across patients? Are stages in the process of recovery perhaps the mirror image of stages of decompensation? Detailed study of schizophrenic patients' experiences over time is necessary to respond to these questions, but preliminary data suggest that all the answers are "yes."[11,24,25] An evolution in recovery through stages of cognitive reorganization accompanied by specific affective stages has been repeatedly described. This sequence appears to be the mirror image of the phases that patients note as leading up to a psychotic episode.

But detailed explorations of these phenomena suggest that there may also be different types of recovery patterns for different types of patients. Recovering patients must reconstruct a fragmented sense of self and purpose. Experientially, it is important to some patients that they have a sense of mastery—achieved, they feel, by understanding the psychotic symptoms and their origins. Others experience the phenomenon of psychotic disorder as alien and try to ignore, deny, or forget it. Still other patients during recovery feel as though they are emerging from a crisis, the end point of which is still unclear. They may experience an anxious uncertainty coupled with a hope that personal growth can occur. Guilt over acts and impulses, grief over loss of psychotic enthrallment, depression, detachment, and a realistic apprehension are emotions frequently described.

Sometimes in recovery a developmental process does appear to be restarted, and severe psychological constraints are painfully and slowly diminished. Perceval[26] and others have described how basic feelings regarding experiences and relationships may be recognized and expressed for the first time in one's life when disturbed cognition and perception diminish. Even for persons who appear to grow as part of their psychotic episode, however, a vulnerability may remain and symptoms recur.[17,27,28] Understandably, this can be a shattering blow to the patient's self-esteem, and clinicians have the difficult task of valuing and working therapeutically with subjective experiences without implying that understanding, integration, and psychological growth create invulnerability. It is in the recovery phase especially that meaningful connections are often misconstrued by patient and clinician to account totally for etiology of illness.

CAUTIONARY NOTES

The richness of the experiential world of some schizophrenic patients provides unique glimpses of unconscious and primitive psychological phenomena and of sequential processes in disorder. But that richness may also lead the patient and clinician into a misleading and antitherapeutic enthrallment. A few caveats will illustrate.

1. Interesting associations often become unquestioned "causal" connections when a theoretical framework (or even common sense) is applied. A patient's impression that psychotic symptoms were precipitated by a job loss may make sense to one clinician. Another clinician, however, might conclude that the loss of a job was the first evidence of disorder in someone biologically vulnerable to overarousal from an endogenous source. At present, the clinician who attempts to understand the patient's experience is in a good position for hypothesis generation but in a poor position to deny or confirm etiological theory. Current trends to deemphasize or ignore the detailed experiences of schizo-

phrenic patients were criticized early in this chapter. However, there is also the danger of ascribing a dazzling or magical quality to what may be incorrect or misleading impressions.

2. The subjective side of schizophrenia is variable between patients and, over time, in the individual. For this reason, one cannot safely speak of the inner life of "schizophrenia."

3. Drawing conclusions about schizophrenic experiences from autobiographical written reports can be misleading. Although these descriptions may be illuminating, many pitfalls exist as well. For one thing, the professional reader is often left unsatisfied concerning the diagnosis. Even when the experiences described are convincingly psychotic, it may not be clear that the writer was schizophrenic. Secondly, autobiographical written reports reflect an unrepresentative sample of experiences. It is a human proclivity to write (and read) about interesting rather than banal phenomena; hence, the more provocative and colorful descriptions will receive the attention. Finally, information on certain types of patients may be totally absent from such reports. To write about psychosis as a personal experience requires motivation, a sense of purpose, a gift for communication, and other attributes often impaired in schizophrenic patients, especially those with process schizophrenia. Do patients with flat affect write telling accounts of their experience? Descriptions of such disorders usually come from clinicians and family members, and even then some degree of inference regarding the patient's experience is necessary.

4. Insights achieved during psychosis may be less valuable than they seem. Insights can occur because unconscious associative processes are prominent, the restraints of logic and social acceptance are lessened, or the patient is sensitive to cues and stimuli that are ordinarily ignored. In any case, the patient and clinician impressed with the opportunity to make meaningful connections may overestimate the therapeutic value of insights, especially if these are not applied to daily behavior in ordinary living situations.

5. Clinicians working therapeutically and intensively with disordered experience may develop a strong sense that they are dealing with the "core of illness." This claim may be more compelling than consideration of a narrow range of descriptive characteristics (e.g., hospital status, illness duration, special psychotic symptoms) as representing the "core." But it is still misleading, because at this time the conceptual core of

schizophrenia has not yet been demonstrated. What is considered to be central in the illness depends on a value judgment. For one viewer, the ability to live in the community may be central; for another, the capacity for pleasure; and for a third, the primacy of certain symptoms.

In spite of these limitations, the detailed study of patient experiences has several practical benefits. Beyond the value of phenomenology *per se*, it is important in many aspects of treatment and in generating hypotheses for research. Furthermore, psychotic experiences, like other personal crises, can generate perspective and conflict resolution and may even promote psychological growth. This is not to glamorize or advocate psychosis, but simply to note the opportunity that may exist when psychosis is conceptualized as having growth-inducing potential.

SUMMARY

The detailed experiential aspects of schizophrenia are important to the patient and have broad implications for treatment and research. Familiarity with the patient's inner world serves as a basis for empathy, and the data gained may define processes involved in onset and recovery. The variety of phenomena described, the failure of some kinds of patients to give such reports, and questions of diagnosis are potential problems requiring consideration in drawing inferences from schizophrenic experiences. The hypotheses generated from intimate knowledge of these experiences may be compelling, but the clinician and investigator must attend to meaningful connections without necessarily assuming that those connections demonstrate causal processes.

RECOMMENDED READING

Kaplan, B. (ed.). *The inner world of mental illness*. New York: Harper & Row, 1964.
Searles, H. The source of anxiety in paranoid schizophrenia. In: *Collected Papers*. New York: International Universities Press, 1965.
Greene, H. *I never promised you a rose garden*. New York: Harper & Row, 1964.
Sechehaye, M. *Autobiography of a schizophrenic girl*. New York: Grune & Stratton, 1951.

REFERENCES

1. Jaspers, K. *General psychopathology* (1923). Translated by J. Hoenig and M. Hamilton. Manchester, England: Manchester University Press, 1963.
2. Freud, S. *Introductory lectures in psychoanalysis.* New York: Boni & Liveright, 1920.
3. Sechehaye, M. *Autobiography of a schizophrenic girl.* New York: Grune & Stratton, 1951.
4. Jefferson, L. I am crazy wild this minute. In: *The inner world of mental illness,* Kaplan, B. (ed.). New York: Harper & Row, 1964.
5. Jung, C. G. The content of the psychoses. In: *Collected Works,* Vol. 3. New York: Pantheon Books, 1953.
6. Fromm-Reichmann, F. *Principles of intensive psychotherapy.* Chicago: University of Chicago Press, 1950.
7. Searles, H. *Collected papers on schizophrenia and related subjects.* New York: International Universities Press, 1965.
8. Sullivan, H. S. *Conceptions of modern psychiatry.* New York: Norton, 1940.
9. Will, O. Comments on the "elements" of schizophrenia, psychotherapy, and the schizophrenic person. In: *The psychotherapy of schizophrenia,* Strauss, J. S., Bowers, M. B., Downey, T. W. *et al.* (eds.). New York: Plenum, 1980.
10. Freedman, B. J. The subjective experience of perceptual and cognitive disturbances in schizophrenia: A review of autobiographical accounts. *Archives of General Psychiatry,* 1974, 30:330–340.
11. Bowers, M. *Retreat from sanity.* New York: Human Sciences Press, 1974.
12. Henry, J. *Pathways to madness.* New York: Random House, 1965.
13. McGlashan, T., and Carpenter, W. Affective symptoms and the diagnosis of schizophrenia. *Schizophrenia Bulletin,* 1979, 5:547–553.
14. Herz, M., and Melville, C. Relapse in schizophrenia. *American Journal of Psychiatry,* 1980, 137:801–805.
15. Strauss, J. S., Gabriel, K. R., Kokes, R. F., Ritzler, B. A., VanOrd, A., and Tarana, E. Do psychiatric patients fit their diagnoses? Patterns of symptomatology as described with the biplot. *Journal of Nervous and Mental Disease,* 1979, 167:105–113.
16. Strauss, J. S. Hallucinations and delusions as points on continua function: Rating scale evidence. *Archives of General Psychiatry,* 1969, 31:581–586.
17. McDonald, N. Living with schizophrenia. In: *The inner world of mental illness,* Kaplan, B. (ed.). New York: Harper and Row, 1964.
18. Krim, S. The insanity bit. In: *The inner world of mental illness,* Kaplan, B. (ed.). New York: Harper & Row, 1964.
19. Anonymous. On being diagnosed schizophrenic. *Schizophrenia Bulletin,* 1976, 2:302–316.
20. Wadeson, H., and Carpenter, W. T., Jr. Subjective experience of schizophrenia. *Schizophrenia Bulletin,* 1976, 2:302–316.
21. Chapman, J. The early symptoms of schizophrenia. *British Journal of Psychiatry,* 1966, 112:225–251.

22. Sartre, J.-P. *La nausée.* Paris: Gallimard, 1937.
23. Freeman, A. M., and Melges, F. T. Depersonalization and temporal disintegration in acute mental illness. *American Journal of Psychiatry,* 1977, 134:679–681.
24. Sachs, M., Carpenter, W. T., Jr., and Strauss, J. S. Recovery from delusions: Three phases documented by patients' interpretation of research procedures. *Archives of General Psychiatry,* 1974, 30:117–120.
25. Docherty, J., VanKammen, D., Siris, S., and Marder, S. Stages of onset of schizophrenic psychoses. *American Journal of Psychiatry,* 1978, 135:420–426.
26. Perceval, J. Narrative of the treatment experienced by a gentleman during a state of mental derangement. In: *The inner world of mental illness,* Kaplan, B. (ed.). New York: Harper & Row, 1964.
27. Leff, J. P., Hirsch, S. R., Gaind, R., Rohde, P. D., and Stevens, B.S. Life events and maintenance therapy in schizophrenic relapse. *British Journal of Psychiatry,* 1973, 123:659–660.
28. Brown, G. W., Birley, J. L. T., and Wing, J. K. Influence of family life on the course of schizophrenic disorders: A replication. *British Journal of Psychiatry,* 1972, 121:241–258.

CHAPTER 5

Prognosis

What is to be the fate of our adolescent patient? He has, after all, characteristic symptoms of schizophrenia, and we have made the preliminary diagnosis based on the information at hand. Even early in the evaluation process, the clinician must make initial treatment plans, and the patient and family need the clinician's perspective in establishing expectations for their future. Considering prognosis is of tantamount importance, and witting and unwitting communications concerning the patient's future begin early in the clinical contact.

The anxiety and misunderstanding surrounding madness is immense, and the worst is often feared. These fears are easily reinforced accidentally by clinicians; hence, patients and families require education concerning the prognostic implications of various components of the illness picture. During one follow-up interview, for example, a patient's mother reported that she had been told her son would never be normal again. On further questioning, we learned that the doctor had indicated that her son's problems were partly genetic and had reassured her that his condition was not the direct result of her parenting. She was, in fact, somewhat reassured but later concluded that, because the disease was genetic, recovery was impossible.

This fatalistic view of schizophrenia was probably not shared by her son's doctor, but it has been shared by many influential psychiatrists. This view was reinforced for many years by the practice of sequestering mental patients in custodial institutions that provided an ambience of hopelessness. The extent to which such a view is justified has been the subject of intensive clinical investigation during the past 20 years, the results of which will be summarized following a brief discussion of the concept of prognosis and its relationship to disease entities.

THE CONCEPT OF PROGNOSIS

Prognosis can be viewed from two vantage points. The first is the natural history concept of disease, the view that the prognosis of a disorder is essentially inherent in the disorder itself. In measles, for example, the succession of events is more or less fixed: fever, then rash, then resolution within about ten days. For such disorders, the importance of their natural history is clear. Establishing the diagnosis enables the physician to tell the patient and family what to expect, and it provides a baseline against which to measure complications and treatment effectiveness. This model is often applied to schizophrenia, and it has been widely believed that a properly made diagnosis of schizophrenia, in and of itself, is predictive of the course of illness.

The second concept of prognosis is more complex and, in practice, more flexible. Course of illness is not viewed as fixed by something intrinsic to the disease but rather is seen as a complex interaction over time between disease and other factors. We have described one such interactional model of disease in an earlier chapter. Prognosis from this point of view may include prior personality, the social context in which the disease develops, factors intrinsic to the disease itself, and the social consequences of illness. From this vantage point, predicting the course of the disorder requires information beyond that necessary for establishing a diagnosis.

The crucial question is the extent to which prognosis is determined by the disorder or can be measurably influenced by a variety of nondiagnostic factors. The outcome may be variable within either frame of reference, since characteristics such as severity of illness could be predictive, even when course and outcome are considered intrinsic to the disease itself. However, the broader concept of prognosis implies a significantly greater heterogeneity in outcome functioning for any given disorder. These points are basic to understanding prognostic views regarding schizophrenia, a brief review of which will be presented next to provide background for understanding the current status of predicting outcome for the individual patient.

VIEWS OF PROGNOSIS IN SCHIZOPHRENIA

The impact of a schizophrenic patient's deterioration, when it occurs, is devastating to patients and their families and friends and striking to physicians. Without doubt, it was such an impact that influenced Kraepelin, who used deteriorating course to validate the concept of dementia praecox. But he also noted that some patients actually had favorable outcomes. There are authorities today who believe that recovery is incompatible with a diagnosis of schizophrenia and many more who consider that the diagnosis implies deteriorating course and poor outcome for most patients. However, in recent years considerable variability in the course of illness has been documented from both clinical and research experiences. This heterogeneity of outcome requires explanation.

Three general types of explanation for variation in the course of schizophrenia have been offered. First is the argument that schizophrenia is a disease of poor prognosis and that recovery or good outcome is sufficient evidence to challenge the diagnosis. Proponents of this explanation suggest that diagnostic errors are made because the wrong criteria are used and/or because there is another disorder (e.g., schizophreniform psychosis) that is easy to confuse with "true" schizophrenia.

The second explanation for the extensive variability in the course of schizophrenia is founded on the belief that schizophrenia is a syndrome comprised of more than one disease entity. The overlapping concepts of poor/good premorbid, process/reactive, or poor/good prognosis subtypes are commonly used subclassifications of schizophrenia, all suggesting that there are two or more types of true schizophrenia with different courses of illness. In all instances, these subtypes require defining criteria besides schizophrenic symptoms. Such characteristics include social behavior in childhood, pre-illness social function, mode of symptom onset, family patterns of illness, and type of affective function. It is possible to describe these variables and their corresponding prognostic implications either dichotomously (supporting a multiple-subtype/disease entity concept) or on a continuum (maintaining a unitary concept of schizophrenia). Current genetic, biochemical, and psychophysiological evidence does not yet provide a definitive basis for choosing between these two concepts.

The third explanation for extensive heterogeneity of outcome in schizophrenia is based on the multidimensional conception of outcome functioning. For many years, it was assumed implicitly that the main aspects of outcome, level of care requirements, and capacity for intrapsychic and social functioning were different facets of a unitary dimension. That is, in the course of schizophrenia these various factors would be closely related to each other. However, recent investigations challenge this assumption, and it seems likely that the various attributes that have been considered as comprising course of illness operate as loosely linked systems, each with its own set of determinants. The finding that a patient may be doing very well in one domain while deteriorating in another confuses the picture and requires a reconceptualization of earlier descriptions of course of illness where outcome was viewed in unitary terms. There is evidence that the multidimensional view of outcome may also hold for other psychiatric disorders besides schizophrenia and provide an important basis for understanding the course of psychopathology in general.

Before discussing the various aspects of outcome and their prediction in more detail, it is important to note that the three points of view discussed above are obviously not mutually exclusive. Nor do any of these views preclude the possibility that the course of illness has become increasingly heterogeneous over time because of less rigid social expectations of deterioration and the impact of more effective treatment. In any case, it is now clear that the diagnosis of schizophrenia based on cross-sectional symptomatology—no matter how stringent—fails to predict outcome in the individual patient. The clinician must incorporate a broad range of data in making prognostic judgments, and aspects of outcome functioning are relatively discrete so that good predictors for one domain may be weak predictors for another. Finally, as we shall make clear later in this chapter, the clinician and patient must realize the limitations of our prognostic capabilities, especially during the early phases of illness.

But how can a prognostic judgment be constructed? It is to this task that we turn next.

SELECTION OF OUTCOME AND PROGNOSTIC VARIABLES

Real patients do not have "an" outcome. One patient with continuous hallucinations may be fully employed, while another patient, unable to function outside of the home, may take extensive responsibility in family affairs. Patients readmitted to the hospital may not be having a symptom relapse as much as a serious break in social function following a stressful event. Some discharged patients are not readmitted to hospitals and may mistakenly be assumed to have a good treatment outcome when, in fact, they are living a vegetative existence with severe dysfunction in a nonhospital setting. These types of outcome situation have been reflected in several recent studies that demonstrate an independence of various outcome processes.[1-3] In the past, the use of a global outcome judgment may have provided the clinician with an opportunity to synthesize the broad range of information concerning outcome functioning into one variable, but it also had the unfortunate effect of suggesting that such a conceptualization is a fully adequate representation of reality.

Thus recent research and clinical experience have demonstrated that assessment of outcome involves sampling from the broad range of human functioning vulnerable to being affected in schizophrenic illness. And, to some extent at least, these areas of function must be considered separately. In the assessment of outcome, symptom type, symptom duration, and hospital status are three obviously important characteristics. One subgroup of symptoms of particular note is what has been called a deficit syndrome, characteristics such as apathy, anhedonia, and loss of curiosity or spontaneity. Of equal importance to symptoms and hospitalization are two other features, social relationships and work functioning. Thus, in all, five basic features must be included in the assessment of outcome in schizophrenia.

When outcome is recognized as involving such a range of relatively independent areas representing multiple processes, it becomes necessary for the prognostician to utilize a multidimensional approach to predicting these outcomes. This consideration, plus extensive evidence, provides the basis for selecting predictor characteristics. In fact, the clinical investigation of prognostic variables has produced surprisingly consistent results, and our present basis for predicting outcome has stood the test of time, study, and common sense.

In selecting predictor variables, nothing is more reasonable than the supposition that prior functioning in any particular domain is likely to be the best predictor of future functioning in that domain. This supposition has been supported by considerable evidence.[4] When patient and family wish to know the likelihood of future hospitalizations, history of previous hospitalizations is most informative. If they wish to know the types of symptoms to anticipate in future episodes, the type of symptomatology in previous episodes is most informative. If they wish to know the social relations and work prognosis, then a careful assessment of prior social and work functioning provides the best information. Recent data from systematic studies suggest that these common sense views are, in fact, valid.[4] Thus, four characteristics are among the most consistently important predictor variables in schizophrenia. These are symptom type, duration of previous psychiatric hospitalization, previous level of social relations function, and previous level of work function. A fifth characteristic, previous duration of symptoms, is probably the best predictor of future symptom duration.

OTHER PROGNOSTIC VARIABLES

Besides the characteristics described above in the multidimensional view of prognosis, several other predictor variables have also been demonstrated as associated at least generally with outcome in schizophrenia. Related to good prognosis are: acute onset of symptomatic episodes, the presence of stressful precipitating factors, quick and relatively full recovery from any illness episode, presence of affective symptomatology, and family history of affective disorders. Characteristics associated with poor prognosis are the opposite: insidious onset, incomplete recovery between episodes, absence of affective symptomatology, presence of blunted or flattened affect, absence of precipitating factors, and a developmental picture suggesting neurological or psychological complications of development. Low IQ and never having been married are also associated with poor outcome.

Many predictors have social and cultural significance and may not be applied with equal validity in all cultures or all socioeconomic classes. Some predictors change with time; for example, marital status is probably less important as a predictor today than it was 30 years ago. Other predictors are difficult to define reliably, even though they appear important conceptually. The presence of precipitating factors, for instance, is often far more difficult to judge than one would anticipate. Psychotic patients tend to have upsetting things occurring in their lives, and it is often difficult to determine the extent to which a stressful event contributes to psychosis or is caused by it. Similarly, affective disturbance is so common in the early stages of psychotic illness that the presence of affective symptomatology may have less prognostic significance than is often believed. There is even some evidence to suggest that affective symptoms are lost if the disorder continues, so that absence of these symptoms may be more a marker than a predictor of chronicity.

HOW SHOULD A PROGNOSIS BE GENERATED?

Once the key outcome and predictor variables have been identified, how can they be used to generate a prognostic judgment? We believe the core of such a judgment should be based on the five predictors (symptom type, symptom duration, duration of previous hospitalization, previous level of social relations function, and previous level of work function) and the five outcome characteristics (future symptom type, future symptom duration, future hospitalization, future social relations, and future work). As noted earlier, each of the predictor variables is generally the best predictor of its corresponding outcome measure; however, there is some crossover as well. A very approximate predictive estimate of global outcome can be generated by summing the four quantitative predictors (all the variables except symptom type).

Conceptually, because of the association between corresponding predictor and outcome variables, we recommend viewing the prognosis/outcome processes as open-linked systems of functioning. Each process (e.g., social relations) has its own continuity over time as well as some interaction with other longitudinal processes. The understanding of these processes and their relationships requires further investigation, but viewing prognosis as involving open-linked systems provides a basic framework for examining and dealing with factors crucial in determining course of illness.

The role of the prognostic variables other than those in the "basic five" multidimensional system described above is somewhat more questionable. Several of them, such as marital status, are subsumed in the multidimensional system (e.g., under previous social relationships); others, as we noted earlier, are difficult to assess reliably. In general, however, we would recommend that the additional prognostic variables be considered as helpful but ancillary to the multidimensional system.

PROGNOSIS AND THE INDIVIDUAL PATIENT

In the discussion thus far, we have been considering some of the major predictor variables and illustrating the inherent complexity in prognostication. We chose factors that have already been subjected to study, but the clinician must weigh much more information when formulating prognosis for any particular patient. What can we say, then, about the young patient we are following from chapter to chapter? As suggested by the earlier discussions, the first step in prognosticating for the individual patient should be to specify that which is being predicted. Specifically, the available information suggests the following:

In terms of predicting symptom duration and future hospitalization, we can make the following estimates. If the symptoms have a recent onset (and especially if the patient has never been previously hospitalized), there is a 30% or greater chance that he will recover completely from his symptoms and not require further hospitalization. There is also a 30% chance that he will fail to show substantial symptomatic improvement. In terms of predicting future symptom type, if the patient does have a symptom remission followed by a recurrence, it is likely that the second episode will be marked by the same symptoms as the first.[5,6]

In regard to the other aspects of prognosis, additional data are important for an optimal predictive estimate. If our patient has a history of poor social relationships marked by withdrawal and absence of friends, he is likely to continue having similar problems—the past predicts the future! Finally, for predicting his future work function—the same principle applies—, past work function is most important.

In the discussion above, we have emphasized that prediction in any specific area of functioning should be founded on a careful review of prior functioning in that area. In attempting to provide some global estimate of outcome, it is clearly necessary to include assessment of multiple dimensions of prior functioning. The "basic five" mentioned earlier provide an important foundation in such an effort. Besides these, for the individual patient the clinician will be able to consider an even larger number of variables, some of which, such as particular types of stress, may be important only to that patient and not generalizable to others.

But even with the most information at our disposal, how good an estimate are we actually able to make? Certainly not good enough to say, "This person will never recover," nor do we have any basis for certainty that a patient will recover and never be troubled again. As a patient is followed over time, we can increase the ability to predict his or her future course, but a healthy degree of uncertainty must always remain. Manfred Bleuler, in an intensive study of schizophrenic patients over a 25-year period, found many chronically, severely disabled patients who improved after having reached a deteriorated state.[7] Most estimates[8,9] suggest that about 20% of variance (a measure of variability) of outcome from the worst possible to the best possible can be predicted by the most effective measures available. Because this is certainly well beyond chance, the predictive power of the characteristics mentioned above is valuable both practically and theoretically. But it is even more important to remember that the current capacity to predict the course of disorder for any particular patient is limited.

In the discussion so far, following general tradition, and the need to simplify somewhat, we have described prognosis in the sense of the "natural history of disorder." The clinician attempting to prognosticate must also weigh the likelihood that treatment will alter the course of illness. This issue will be discussed at length in the chapters on treatment, but a few considerations should be mentioned here. In general, our discussion on prognosis relates to the course of illness in the context of current "average" treatments. It will be obvious that for a patient judged to be a good responder to pharmacotherapy, the prognosis will vary depending on the clinician's estimate of a likelihood of compliance with treatment recommendations. Analogous principles hold for other treatments. As new methods of treatment are introduced or the integration of multiple treatments leads to greater efficacy, prognostication will have to pay greater attention to the specific capacities to alter course of illness with therapeutic intervention.

WHAT HAS BECOME OF SCHIZOPHRENIC DETERIORATION?

The considerable variation in the outcome of schizophrenia noted earlier appears at least partly to be a function of variations in the factors comprising the multidimensional model of prognosis. How, then, did some of the earlier views of predictable deterioration come about? Partly because of sampling. The patients most readily available to the clinicians who first defined schizophrenia were mostly institutionalized and chronic. As the availability of psychiatrists and treatment has increased, more patients are seen who have recently become ill and hence include the most hopeful cases. It may be these recent-onset patients with characteristic symptoms of schizophrenia and favorable outcome who have forced us to seek explanations for the wide range of prognosis that exists.

A second possibility for the need to reevaluate the concept of schizophrenic deterioration is that earlier and more effective treatment combined with efforts to minimize the chronicity-inducing effects of psychiatric hospitals may have altered the course of schizophrenia. The decline of treatment involving prolonged isolation of the patient from family, friends, and community is one important factor, reducing the likelihood of deterioration.[10,11] Prolonged institutionalization of any kind tends to dampen motivation and lead to the degeneration of coping and social skills. The extent of change in hospital treatment may be hard to realize unless one recalls the commonplace situation of even fifteen years ago, when patients were often dressed only in hospital pajamas and bathrobes, their letters were censored or not permitted, visitors were severely restricted, and the only treatment generally available was inpatient care in centers often located twenty miles or more from patients' homes, making visiting difficult, if not impossible.

In the past several years, community-oriented treatment, psychotropic medication, and increased respect for the human needs and abilities of schizophrenic inpatients have played a significant role in reversing earlier treatment practices. With these newer approaches, it has been possible for patients to be treated increasingly as individuals in a community context, often living with their families and maintaining useful occupational roles during the treatment process. In some instances, the tendency to keep disordered patients in the community has become a dogma dominated by the lower cost of such care or by insensitivity to problems that excesses in the practice can generate involving adverse impact on the community, on the family, and, of course, on the patient. In general, however, earlier identification of disorder and more effective community-based treatment practices have contributed to the revision of the grave prognosis that once automatically accompanied the diagnosis of schizophrenia.

IMPLICATIONS OF THE REVISED PROGNOSTIC ESTIMATES

There are several very practical implications of recognizing variability in the course of schizophrenia and the current status of prognostic estimates.

1. As clinicians, we must live with, and help our patients live with, considerable uncertainty about their future and their response to treatment. This uncertainty is more valid than the overt and covert negative expectations so often associated with the diagnosis of schizophrenia.

2. We must be extraordinarily cautious in trying to establish cause-and-effect relationships for individual patients. Impressions of treatment efficacy, complicated in themselves, must be further tempered by considering the patient's prognostic status as well as unexplained prognostic variability. For example, common statements such as "patients treated early in the disorder are more likely to recover" need to be received with the understanding that any patient "early" in the disorder, that is, where there is not a history of chronicity, is more likely to recover—with or without treatment—than a patient in whose case chronicity is a demonstrated part of the illness.

3. In research comparing treatment approaches, interpretation of results requires a comprehensive view of patients' prognostic status.

4. Estimates of treatment responsiveness must be incorporated into prognostic judgments by clinicians.

What, then, is the prognosis of schizophrenia? Schizophrenia is a severe illness, and many patients so diagnosed manifest extensive mental and personality dysfunction throughout their lives. Others recover. Every imaginable variation between full recovery and devastation occurs. The prediction of where in this range a particular patient or group of patients is likely to fall can be improved by considering the characteristics described in this chapter.

SUMMARY

Originally, the prognosis of schizophrenia was considered to involve deterioration and to preclude total recovery. As more careful studies have been carried out with objective rating scales and diagnostic criteria and with more representative samples of patients, diverse outcomes from complete recovery to deterioration have been demonstrated.

The multidimensional view of prognosis involving special attention to the predictive importance of areas of premorbid adjustment demonstrates that the course and outcome of schizophrenia, although sometimes involving chronicity, is a complex set of processes, symptom types, prior duration of symptoms and hospitalization, level of social relationships, and level of work function, each of which needs to be assessed and considered.

RECOMMENDED READING

Bleuler, M. The long-term course of the schizophrenic psychoses. *Psychological Medicine*, 1974, 4:244–254.
Strauss, J. S., and Carpenter, W. T., Jr. Prediction of outcome in schizophrenia. III. Five-year outcome and its predictors. *Archives of General Psychiatry*, 1977, 34:159–163.

REFERENCES

1. Kenniston, K., Boltax, S., and Almond, R. Multiple criteria of treatment outcome. *Journal of Psychiatric Research*, 1971, 8:107–118.
2. Schwartz, C. C., Myers, J. K., and Astrachan, B. M. Concordance of multiple assessments of the outcome of schizophrenia. *Archives of General Psychiatry*, 1975, 32:1221–1227.
3. Strauss, J. S., and Carpenter, W. T., Jr. Prediction of outcome in schizophrenia. I. Characteristics of outcome. *Archives of General Psychiatry*, 1972, 27:739–746.
4. Strauss, J. S., and Carpenter, W. T., Jr. Prediction of outcome in schizophrenia. II. Relationships between predictor and outcome variables. *Archives of General Psychiatry*, 1974, 31:37–42.
5. Babigian, H., Gardner, E., Miles, H., and Romano, J. Diagnostic consistency and change in a follow-up study of 1215 patients. *American Journal of Psychiatry*, 1965, 121:895–901.
6. World Health Organization. *Schizophrenia: An international follow-up study*. New York: Wiley, 1979.
7. Bleuler, M. The long-term course of the schizophrenic psychoses. *Psychological Medicine*, 1974, 4:244–254.
8. Brown, G., Bone, M., Dalison, B., and Wing, J. *Schizophrenia and social care*. London: Oxford University Press, 1966.
9. Strauss, J. S., and Carpenter, W. T., Jr. Prediction of outcome in schizophrenia. III. Five-year outcome and its predictors. *Archives of General Psychiatry*, 1977, 34:159–163.
10. Barton, R. *Institutional neurosis*. Bristol: Wright, 1959.
11. Wing, J. and Brown, G. *Institutionalism and schizophrenia*. Cambridge: Cambridge University Press, 1970.

CHAPTER 6

The Extent of the Problem

EPIDEMIOLOGY OF SCHIZOPHRENIA

Epidemiology in mental health focuses on assessing the amount and distribution of mental disorders in the population. Such information provides the means for improving prevention and treatment and serves as a basis for administrative planning.[1] The epidemiologist also examines associations between population characteristics and disorders that may clarify the origins of mental disorders or aid in identifying homogeneous groups of patients. This chapter will describe epidemiological findings in schizophrenia that delineate the extent of the problem and provide information relevant to etiology and pathogenesis from an epidemiological perspective.

Schizophrenia must be recognized as one of the world's major unsolved health problems. It is by no means a rare disease, with an estimated 100,000 new cases receiving care each year (recorded or treated incidence rate of about .5/1,000) in the United States.[3] Community surveys in various countries give estimates of the number of cases at any point of time (point prevalence) ranging from 0.5% to 3.0%. This range reflects variations in diagnostic practices and other methodological differences among studies.

Most workers conclude that the number of individuals diagnosable as having schizophrenia sometime during their lives (life-time prevalence or risk for schizophrenia) is stable from country to country at about .19–.95%, although a broader definition of schizophrenia has at times generated a higher prevalence in the United States.[4] The possibility that real (rather than methodological) differences in incidence or prevalence exist among cultures cannot be excluded at this time, but the similarity of rates is striking, and major culture-bound differences (such as the apparent increased prevalence in Ireland[4]) appear to be rare. Course and content of psychopathology, such as type of delusions and affective picture, do vary somewhat across cultures, of course, but form and frequency of schizophrenia are, to a considerable degree, constant.

In the mid-1970s, it was estimated that 600,000 diagnosed schizophrenics in the United States were actively receiving treatment and that some 62% of these cases would receive hospital care at some point during illness.[2] Minkoff[5] estimates about 1,100,000 cases of schizophrenia in the United States in 1977–1978; and Kramer,[6] studying shifts in size and age distribution of the general population, projects that this number will increase by another 163,000 by 1985.

It must be appreciated that obtaining good, communitywide data on a condition as personal and socially undesirable as psychotic illness is extraordinarily difficult; thus, most of the figures cited above may almost routinely underestimate the extent of illness by omission of cases not receiving treatment, by exclusion of mild or covert forms of illness, and by suppression or falsification of relevant data by those responding to survey questionnaires or interviews. There is also evidence that clinicians tend selectively to under-diagnose schizophrenia in certain demographic groups, such as in upper-class patients.

Despite the steady rise in cases based on population increases, the number of hospitalized schizophrenic patients has been dramatically reduced since 1950. The deinstitutionalization movement, characterized by efforts to curb chronic institutional care and to enhance community-based treatment, and made feasible as a large-scale effort by the introduction of antipsychotic drugs, has produced some of the most remarkable statistics in health care outside the conquests of infectious diseases. In 1955, the large state mental hospitals had a resident population (largely schizophrenic) of 558,922. Twenty years after that peak year, in 1975, in spite of considerable increase in the general population, there were 365,000 fewer patients residing in those facilities[7]; and by 1977 the figure was reduced by another 23,000.[8] Although this process was aided by increased short-term inpatient facilities in community hospitals and increased use of nursing homes for chronic patients, not all of the changes are attributable to these alternative inpatient facilities.

The reduction in the number of schizophrenic inpatients has now slowed, and further substantial reductions may require important treatment innovations and far greater capacity to provide community support and treatment to chronically impaired discharged patients.

It even seems likely that some increase in the number of hospitalized schizophrenic patients will occur in the future, since many of today's hospital residents represent the hard core of "untreatable" patients, who are not amenable to community-based care. Moreover, future changes in the population's age distribution will sharply increase the number of schizophrenic patients in need of treatment by increasing that part of the population at risk. Finally, if community-based efforts result in better case identification and linkage of services, fewer patients will "fall through the cracks," and hospitals may begin to serve a larger proportion of those in need of inpatient care.

At the same time that the resident population of state hospitals has been decreasing, the number of admissions to these facilities has risen. In the two decades from 1955–1975, admissions more than doubled, increasing from 152,286 to 376,156.[7] Most of these admissions were readmissions; in 1975, 69% of all admissions to state mental hospitals had received prior psychiatric inpatient care.[9]

Considered together, the statistics presented here, even with the shifting patterns of care, indicate that schizophrenia is a common, severe illness and that it is characterized by continuing treatment needs. The importance of the problem is further highlighted by recalling that many patients have chronic disabilities beginning in adolescence or early adulthood and anticipated long life spans; the burden of illness for many individuals, therefore, may last over 50 years.

Another vantage point from which to view the scope of an illness is to consider the financial cost. Exact figures are not available, but the large number of patients being treated and the extensive use of hospitals for their care drives direct treatment cost for schizophrenia into the billions (perhaps $17 billion per year).[10] Indirect costs, staggering when one estimates the years of unemployment, required support for housing, food and necessities, training, facilities development, supplemental and other hidden expenses, probably raises the monetary burden of schizophrenic illness close to $40 billion per year.[10]

When viewed from the perspective of the extent of suffering and disability in such a large number of people, the quality and quantity of resources available for patient care and research are shamefully low. For example, the direct and indirect cost of schizophrenia may surpass costs of cancer, but schizophrenia research cannot even claim a respectable fraction of the resources available for the "war on cancer." Furthermore, from a strictly financial point of view, advances in treating schizophrenia potentially save money rather than simply requiring more expensive care. A work program which can reduce the unemployment rate from two-thirds to one-half will generate an enormous reduction in the indirect cost of illness. This contrasts with many other severe illnesses for which new therapies are expensive and prolong life (thereby prolonging duration and cost of treatment). These facts are relevant to administrative and political funding considerations; but to the clinician, patient, family, and, to some extent, society, the well-being of the sick individual is the preeminent consideration making the dearth of resources available especially tragic.

Many factors contribute to the disparity between needed and available resources, but the social stigma associated with schizophrenia is one of the most important. The conditions of hospital care have often been shameful, conditions which would be unthinkable in the case of, say, cardiac patients. The deinstitutionalization movement has been seized by a combination of apathy and politics; using it to save money, therefore, has become as important as enhancing care, and thousands of patients have been neglected by the health system as they are sent to communities unprepared for their treatment. We cannot imagine that increased feasibility of ambulatory care for patients with renal failure could lead to the closing of hospital-based hemodialysis units without providing the required community-based facilities. But the exact analogy has occurred in many states as psychiatric hospital facilities were reduced without providing a feasible community treatment and support alternative.

The disparity between need and resources reflects, among other things, the disenfranchised social status of the severely mentally ill.[11] The stigma of madness and the debilitation of illness combine to preclude public advocacy on behalf of schizophrenia. We annually witness the dramatic effects of well-known public figures affected by cancer, alcoholism, and neurological diseases leading the fight for research and treatment resources. Because of its early onset and associated social disabilities, schizophrenia is underrepresented at the "top." Because of the stigma (and an understandable wish for privacy), we see few public figures pointing to the tragedy of schizophrenic illness in their families.

EPIDEMIOLOGICAL FINDINGS IN POPULATION SUBGROUPS

A number of epidemiological findings suggest that certain subgroups are particularly vulnerable to schizophrenia. We will comment on a few of these to illustrate the implications of such data for understanding etiology.

Schizophrenia is more prevalent in certain population groups, such as those of lower socioeconomic status. Such pooling may result from social and/or genetic etiological factors, and/or it may be a consequence of illness. This latter possibility is most compelling, and is most aptly stated as the downward drift hypothesis of Faris and Dunham.[12] These investigators and others have observed that schizophrenic patients migrate toward areas of poverty (e.g., inner cities), drifting down the social class scale. Kohn[13] formulates this social class phenomenon differently, suggesting that conditions in the social structure and experience of lower class persons produce greater stress and less flexible coping mechanisms that may contribute to schizophrenia vulnerability. This provides an etiological view that could be seen as complementing or conflicting with the consequence of illness orientation represented by the social drift hypothesis. The extent to which the etiological view is valid, however, is questioned by those who find that parents of schizophrenics have a normal population class distribution, suggesting that their schizophrenic offspring, in contrast to the case in the general population, fail to rise to higher class status and/or spiral downward once illness begins.[14]

It is also possible that differential migration influencing both genetic distribution and social stress could lead to greater prevalence in some geographic or social class populations. The higher prevalence of schizophrenia found in the children of first generation immigrants, for example, could be explained either by genetic vulnerability or stress hypotheses.[15,16]

Another demographic pattern of schizophrenia is its interesting distribution by age and sex. Overall, schizophrenia occurs equally in males and females. However, males have an earlier onset. The peak age for first admission to hospital in males is between ages 15 and 24, and for females, between ages 25 and 34. This implies that there are important differences in biological, psychological, and/or social factors by sex that affect the occurrence of schizophrenia. It has been suggested, for example, that men face crucial life stresses a decade earlier than females.[17] It is also useful to recall that the subtype paranoid schizophrenia has the latest age of onset and that this subtype is thought to be more common among males. This finding, of course, is not incompatible with the age/sex distribution for schizophrenia generally, since other types of schizophrenia could more than compensate in terms of their age/sex patterns.

During the last decade, several studies have demonstrated that schizophrenics are statistically more likely to be born in the late winter and early spring months. This phenomenon has been observed in both the northern and southern hemispheres.[18] The effect of season of birth on an individual's risk for manifesting schizophrenia may vary with age of onset and sex.[19,20] These epidemiological findings suggest that season of birth is a marker of etiological relevance for a subgroup of patients, but it is not clear whether season of conception, gestation, or birth is the crucial variable.

Viral hypotheses have received renewed credence based on these reports and the discovery of slow-virus illnesses such as Jakob–Creutzfeldt and kuru diseases.[21,22] Viral hypotheses have also been suggested by an interesting question regarding the history of schizophrenia, namely, whether this illness has existed throughout recorded time or only since the nineteenth century. This is relevant to the speculations that schizophrenia may have resulted from a mutation or virus (e.g., smallpox vaccine) and spread worldwide in recent history, not yet reaching geographical areas still isolated from the modern world.

SUMMARY

An epidemiological perspective on schizophrenia demonstrates the magnitude of the problem. A sizable incidence rate together with a considerably higher prevalence level reflecting the problems of chronicity and recurrence are impressive enough. But when these are combined with consideration of the disorder's severity, the scope of the problem is seen as gigantic and dwarfs the resources available for treatment and research. Specific vulnerable subgroups revealed by epidemiological studies suggest especially that social class, age/sex characteristics, and season of birth may have significant etiological implications.

RECOMMENDED READINGS

Babigian, H. M. Schizophrenia: Epidemiology. In: *Comprehensive textbook of psychiatry*, Vol. 3, Kaplan, H. I., Freedman, A. M., and Sadock, B. J. (eds.). Baltimore: Williams and Wilkins, 1980.
Report of the Task Panel on Nature and Scope of the Problems. *Report of the President's Commission on Mental Health*, Vol. 2, 1978, 1–138.

REFERENCES

1. Lillienfeld, A. M. *Foundations of epidemiology.* New York: Oxford Press, 1976.
2. Report of the Task Panel on Nature and Scope of the Problems. *Report of the President's Commission on Mental Health,* Vol. 2, 1978, 1–138.
3. Babigian, H. M. Schizophrenia: Epidemiology. In: *Comprehensive Textbook of Psychiatry,* Vol. 3. Kaplan, H. I., Freedman, A. M., and Sadock, B. J. (eds.). Baltimore: Williams and Wilkins, 1980.
4. Scheper-Highes, N. *Saints, scholars, and schizophrenics.* Berkeley: University of California Press, 1979.
5. Minkoff, K. A map of the chronic mental patient. In: *The chronic mental patient,* Talbott, J. A. (ed.). Washington: American Psychiatric Association, 1978.
6. Kramer, M. *Population changes and schizophrenia, 1970–1975.* Rockville, Maryland: National Institute of Mental Health, 1976.
7. Unpublished data, Division of Biometry and Epidemiology, National Institute of Mental Health.
8. Witkin, M. J. Provisional patient movement and selective administrative data, state and county mental hospitals, inpatient services by state: United States, 1976. Mental Health Statistical Note, No. 153, August 1979.
9. Division of Biometry and Epidemiology, National Institute of Mental Health. Readmission to inpatient services of state and county mental hospitals, United States, 1969, 1973, and 1975. Memorandum No. 32, Rockville, Maryland, February 10, 1978.
10. Report of the Task Panel on Cost and Financing. *Report of the Preesident's Commission on Mental Health,* Vol. 2, 497–544.
11. Bachrach, L. L. Planning mental health services for chronic patients. *Hospital and Community Psychiatry,* June 30, 1979, 387–393.
12. Faris, R. E. L., and Dunham, H. W. *Mental disorders in urban areas: An ecological study of schizophrenia and other psychoses.* Chicago: University of Chicago Press, 1939.
13. Kohn, M. L. Social class and schizophrenia: A critical review and a reformulation. *Schizophrenia Bulletin,* 1973, No. 7 (Winter): 60–79.
14. Hare, E. H., Price, J. S., and Slater, E. Parental social class in psychiatric patients. *British Journal of Psychiatry,* 1972, 121:515–524.
15. Rosenthal, D., Goldberg, I., Jacobsen, B., Wender, P. H., Kety, S. S., Schulsinger, F., and Eldred, C. A. Migration, heredity, and schizophrenia. *Psychiatry,* 1974, 37:321–339.
16. Odegaard, O. Emigration and insanity. *Acta Psychiatrica Scandinavica,* 1932, supplement 4.
17. Lewine, R. W., Strauss, J. S., and Gift, T. E. Sex difference in age of schizophrenia onset: Fact or artifact? *American Journal of Psychiatry,* in press.
18. Dalen, P. *Season of birth in schizophrenia and other mental disorders.* Amsterdam: North Holland Publishing, 1975.
19. Hare, E. H. Variations in the season distribution of births of psychotic patients in England and Wales. *British Journal of Psychiatry,* 1978, 132:155–158.

20. Pulver, A. E. An investigation of the relationship between schizophrenia and season of birth: A differentiation of subgroups. Unpublished thesis, Johns Hopkins University, 1978.
21. Hare, E. H. Schizophrenia as an infectious disease. *British Journal of Psychiatry*, 1979, 135:468–473.
22. Torrey, E. F. Slow and latent viruses in schizophrenia. *Lancet*, 1973, 2:22–24.

CHAPTER 7

Etiologies of Schizophrenia

BIOLOGICAL

INTRODUCTION

A medical model seems inescapable when considering the biological factors that may contribute to schizophrenia. The question is which medical model is most appropriate. An interactive developmental model provides, we believe, a broad conception of disease that is most adequate for integrating the available facts relevant to the etiologies of schizophrenia. However, genetic and biochemical hypotheses have often been presented within a narrower biomedical model of illness. Such a model has stated or implied that deviations in brain physiology are sufficient to account for schizophrenia without the need to implicate environmental factors. In such a view, psychology and sociology are recognized as relevant to the expression of illness, of course, but etiology is viewed solely in biomedical terms. The presumed brain dysfunction could be conceptualized as structural or functional. In either case, etiology might originate within the brain (e.g., in abnormal limbic system anatomy or function), or the brain could be viewed as the organ of response (e.g., to an abnormal metabolite formed in the gut or liver).

Narrow somatic concepts of schizophrenia have often led to simple three-step etiological theories. For example, a mutant gene is viewed as producing a metabolic alteration which then causes symptoms of schizophrenia. Such gene→biochemical→symptom models led a generation of investigators to search for abnormal metabolites and abnormal structures and led many clinicians to assume that somatic interventions were central to treatment, with psychological interventions being either peripheral or totally irrelevant. This orientation of biological psychiatry had its psychological counterpart among those psychiatrists who ignored biology and viewed mental aberrations as essentially psychological phenomena, involving primarily psychological etiologies and treatments.

The biological model described above captures the essence of how biological psychiatry was conceptualized in America from the postwar period until the mid-1960s and was rigidified by the heated polemics between psychophiles and biophiles during that period. The conflict between camps was heightened by the fact that biological psychiatry attracted many neuroscientists who were not trained in the elaborate theories and techniques of interpersonal psychology and often were not clinically experienced with schizophrenic patients. Clinicians often viewed biological theories of schizophrenia as immodest at best and implausible at worst.

On the other hand, of course, many psychiatrists, enthralled with psychoanalytic theory and interpersonal therapies, neglected the brain side of the brain–mind problem. This neglect and the bio–psycho schism was further promoted by the arrogance of many adherents of psychoanalytic theory and related therapies. During the period being discussed, the psychoanalytically trained psychiatrist had greater prestige and influence than his colleague oriented toward social, biological, or eclectic psychiatry. Biological hypotheses could have been wisely criticized from the position of intrapsychic and interpersonal theories, but too often censure, rather than thoughtful criticism, was applied.

Constructive criticism became less likely because enthrallment with abstract and complex interpersonal theory had led most clinicians away from the tedious and frustrating treatment of chronic psychotic patients. There were, of course, some individual and family therapists who continued to work with such patients during this time, but they were the exceptions. These unfortunate circumstances discouraged interest in biological psychiatry among psychologically oriented clinicians and provided an additional impediment to the development of biologically oriented clinical psychiatry.

With sophisticated clinicians offering little help in developing appropriate clinical models for biological inquiry, bold biological proposals and incautious reports were often followed by failures of replication. This sequence was used further to disparage, although it would have been more helpful to view these difficulties as the beginning activity of a fledgling but indispensable field of inquiry.

The integration of metapsychology and brain physiology desired by Freud[1] has not yet occurred, but polarization in psychiatry has lessened. Collaboration across disciplinary lines is firmly established and is often accepted as more constructive than polemics. Modesty of claim and sophistication of method now characterize the leading biological investigations of schizophrenia. The biomedical model continues to be effective for designing biochemical investigations, but biological hypotheses are increasingly set in the framework of a more comprehensive socio-psycho-biomedical model.

Reacting to the successes and impact of biologically and pharmacologically oriented investigators, clinical investigators interested in interpersonal theories are now accepting the rules of clinical science and are beginning to design studies which are potentially informative about the strengths and limitations of psychosocial hypotheses. Some leading psychoanalysts, Searles[2] for instance, pursue a careful phenomenological exploration of schizophrenic patients rather than simply espousing the sweeping etiological theories of the past. Others, notably family theorists such as Wynne and Singer,[3] have taken on the difficult task of specifying and testing complicated clinical hypotheses. Investigators no longer find it necessary to negate one level of theory in order to subscribe to another. The products of this recent evolution will be illustrated in this and the subsequent chapter.

SOME GENERAL CONSIDERATIONS

The Assumption of Biological Cause

Most influential thinkers in the field of schizophrenia have assumed a somatic etiology. This was true of Kraepelin, Bleuler, and Freud and is no less true of most workers today. Although the supposition, especially if modified to fit into a biopsychosocial model, is reasonable, plausible, and attractive, it is important to realize that somatic etiology is often assumed in the face of otherwise inexplicable psychopathology, even without supporting evidence. Following psychological principles, Bleuler[4] felt that loosening of associations could give rise to other manifestations of schizophrenia, but loosening of associations was the irreducible factor that could not be accounted for on psychological grounds. Therefore, somatic etiology was assumed. Freud,[5] believing

that schizophrenic patients were unable to establish a transference relationship, proferred a constitutional etiology to explain this incapacity.

Etiological assumptions are not always made in this direction; in
other disorders, subjective symptoms which cannot be accounted for on
somatic grounds are often presumed to be psychological in origin. An
internist evaluating a patient with head pain will consider several somatic
etiologies. If supporting evidence is not found, it is common practice to
diagnose the pain as psychogenic, even if evidence for psychological
etiology is lacking.

A more neutral and conservative position when considering illness
of undetermined origin is an atheoretical view, making it explicit that
etiology is unknown. Psychogenic headache should be diagnosed on the
basis of positive evidence for psychogenic etiology, as well as from
negative evidence for somatic conditions which could account for the
pain. Tools are not presently available in the study of schizophrenia to
demonstrate definitively its etiology and pathogenesis; hence, it is desirable for the clinician and investigator to maintain interest in the broadest
range of inquiry. The brain is the functional apparatus underlying the
mind. One cannot expect that a disordered mind would fail to be reflected
in brain function, nor could disordered brain function in relevant areas
fail to have concomitant mind manifestations.

Schizophrenia as a Functional Psychosis

Schizophrenia is classified as a functional psychosis. The term is
ambiguous, but we use it to indicate disordered mental functioning in
which etiological factors remain to be determined and a physiological
basis has not been demonstrated. The use of the term *functional* for
schizophrenia began with the failure of neuropathologists to find altered
anatomy to explain the symptoms of schizophrenic patients. *Functional*
does not imply nonorganic, but it does suggest that brain disturbance in
schizophrenia is based on disharmony in neural functioning, rather than
on structural damage.

The present state of the field does not permit final falsification or
verification of this assumption, but there should be little surprise if the
use of ultramicroscopic technology permits the identification of structural
changes at the subcellular level. Neuropathologists have often observed
changes in the brains of schizophrenic patients at autopsy, and
techniques such as the pneumoencephalogram have often shown ab-

normalities. In the past, these reports have been discounted because the findings varied so much from patient to patient, provided no anatomical basis for the particular manifestations of the disease, and could have been artifacts associated with institutional care, chronic illness, trauma, or (more recently) drug effects. However, a recent study using computerized axial tomography reported structural changes in a high proportion of schizophrenic patients and promises to reopen the question of gross anatomic abnormalities in at least a subgroup of schizophrenic patients.[6] Because of improved research methods, there is also renewed interest in the possibility of postmortem examinations revealing neuropathological and biochemical abnormalities.[7]

During recent years, increasing emphasis has been placed on studying biochemical and electrophysiological variables reflecting functioning of the intact brain, rather than on anatomical and postmortem characteristics. The fact that psychoactive drugs act primarily by altering function rather than structure is one compelling argument for these strategies. Although psychoactive drugs may also induce structural changes with long-term exposure, such changes are not implicated in their immediate behavioral effects and seem unlikely to be involved in their therapeutic action.

Multiple Perspectives

In considering possible etiologies of schizophrenia arising from abnormal nervous system function, it is important to view this function in the broadest way, including potentially all aspects of nervous system physiology. It is also important to note that the biology of schizophrenia after the disorder becomes established may be different from the biology of its etiology or pathogenesis. This distinction permits examination of the biological attributes of schizophrenia and suspension of cause–effect judgments until adequate etiological study paradigms are available.

Finally, in considering biological etiologies or any etiological hypothesis, it must be remembered that various orientations are often not mutually exclusive. For example, genetic or viral causes may produce altered protein synthesis, which could be reflected in defective electrophysiological signal processing. The virologist, geneticist, physiologist, and psychologist all could provide an explanatory theory of this process from his or her own vantage. Even the domains of interpersonal communication or responses to stressful life events could be added to this chain, since they too require a biological mechanism. For this reason, all disciplines relevant to schizophrenia share an interest in brain biochemistry. But also because these domains interact, the primacy of causality across bio-, psycho-, and social spheres cannot be assumed. When possible, biological theories of schizophrenia are put forward as postulated biochemical mechanisms, and several such theories will be reviewed below. But in the discussion of models and concepts in the next several paragraphs, the reader should also appreciate the potential variety of cause–effect relationships across conceptual domains.

MODELS OF ETIOLOGY

The Static Model

Different models guide investigations into the biology of schizophrenia. The static model encourages the investigator to identify a unique biological substance or mechanism which induces changes associated with schizophrenia. The search for an abnormal metabolite is typical. Here one assumes that the presence of an abnormal substance causes the manifest psychopathology. The transmethylation hypothesis is the best representative of this conceptual approach and will be described in detail later.

Static models are important for encouraging precision and testability of hypotheses, but they also have major limitations. Many biological variables change in relationship to clinical status. Understanding the temporal sequences of these associations will increase our knowledge of the psychobiology of psychoses, but in the study of etiology and pathogenesis it is crucial to separate factors that are mainly correlates of a clinical state from factors that precede and therefore may cause it. The latter may be linked to basic vulnerability, while factors associated with more transitory states of manifest illness require that their temporal primacy be documented before cause and effect can be assumed. Even when biological change precedes behavioral change, it is possible, of course, that the chain of events may reflect parallel processes rather than etiology.

Static models have generally provided an inadequate frame of reference to account for dynamic interactions across time and across domains of organismic functioning. When postulated abnormalities are confirmed, there has been a tendency to presume that they cause, rather than reflect, psychosis. The cause/concomitant distinction has been underemphasized in this model, and rules for establishing etiological and pathogenic significance have only recently been rigorously applied.[8]

The Dynamic Neurobiologic Model

This model assumes that changes in the interactions between physiological systems (e.g., altered homeostasis) are involved in the biological basis of psychopathology. The model assumes that many variables must be considered to provide a framework for understanding schizophrenia. Not only the quantity of dopamine at synapses, but turnover rate, receptor sensitivity, the status of short- and long-loop feedback mechanisms, the activation of presynaptic receptors, and balance with reciprocal neurotransmitter systems may be involved. A dynamic model has the beneficial effect of encouraging the investigator to identify systems of dysfunction related to schizophrenia, rather than to identify the one variable that causes the disorder. Dynamic concepts also encourage investigators to be circumspect in interpreting results of specific studies, since only a few of many critical variables can be assessed within any experimental design. These models of schizophrenia are likely to be tentative and incomplete when contrasted to the explanatory power of static models, but they appear likely to be more valid, considering the complexity of brain physiology and of schizophrenia.

The Adaptational Model

Adaptational models are a special case of the dynamic model. Both models are similar in assuming multiple, interacting variables, but the adaptational model calls attention to the organism's responses to disruption of homeostasis as well as to the disruption itself. Neurobiological responses aimed at preventing or minimizing dysfunction may "overshoot the mark," and the perseverance or cascading of such adaptive responses may cause further physiological impairment. Seyle[9] described derailments of adaptation leading to disease states, and psychoanalytic theory postulates adaptive functions (defenses) that lead to symptoms including hallucinations and delusions.[10] Adaptation models assume that any step in a chain of biological reactions may be adaptive—an adaptation to an event which may be internal and biochemical, internal and psychological, or external.

The difference in focus of dynamic and adaptive models is illustrated by the pharmacokinetics of antipsychotic medications. Dynamic models foster (but do not require) the assumption that immediate pharmacological consequences are the most important aspect of the therapeutic effect in drug treatment for schizophrenia. An adaptational model, on the other hand, focuses more on the long-range neurobiological adjustment to the effects of these compounds and leads to hypotheses that it is the human system's adaptation to the pharmacological effect that is therapeutic. Except for the rapid control of certain types of symptoms, the time course for therapeutic effect of antipsychotic medications fits an adaptational model more closely than it fits the simpler dynamic model.

TYPES OF BIOLOGICAL ETIOLOGY

Genetic Etiologies

The possibility of genetic etiologies for schizophrenia has long been a focus of interest. Especially in the past, advocacy of this orientation has occupied one pole in the nature/nurture argument. The polemics of the nature/nurture controversy have not proved useful or valid, however, and this dilemma is now generally resolved by considering genetic factors as contributing to the vulnerability to schizophrenia, rather than by viewing schizophrenia as directly caused by abnormal genes. This modified view facilitates an integration of genetic data with social and psychological factors and avoids the limitations of an exclusively genetic etiological theory. It is now appreciated that there ar many intervening variables between genotype and phenotypic expression of complex heritable phenomena such as mental illness. The concept of one or more specifically schizophrenic genotypes may be useful as a point of reference, but it is almost certain that a protein chemist acting alone will never be able to specify those variables which induce or prevent the schizophrenic phenotype.

Genetic models are valuable in that, when considering a particular schizophrenic patient at least, they resolve the chicken/egg dilemma. In determining the role of causal factors in schizophrenia, cause–effect sequences are often obscure, but understandably, for any particular patient, genetic etiology is accepted as coming first.

Because there is ample evidence supporting a genetic component in chronic forms of schizophrenia (and genetic contributions have not been excluded in acute forms), some version of the genetic model is essential to an understanding of the etiology.[11,12] The various twin, family, adoptive, and biochemical studies that indicate a genetic component, however, also provide evidence for genetic heterogeneity and/or nongenetic intervening variables. Patterns of schizophrenia in families are not compatible with any simple mode of genetic transmission; multigene and partial penetrance concepts, therefore, are generally advocated. The higher concordance for illness found in monozygotic compared to dizygotic twins implicates genetic factors, but the high degree of nonconcordance (> 50%) and the dissimilarity in manifest psychopathology between concordant twins suggests the crucial role of environmental influences. Environment is defined broadly in this regard to include possible etiological variables as diverse as intrauterine nutrition and parental communication styles.

Adoptive studies have focused primarily on offspring born to persons with schizophrenia who have been adopted by nonschizophrenic parents, but other parent–child combinations have been studied as well.[13,14] This research has demonstrated increased schizophrenia and schizophrenia spectrum disorders in biological relatives of chronic schizophrenic patients, but not in their adoptive relatives. These same studies also demonstrate the heterogeneity of the genetic component and/or the environmental influences relevant to manifest pathology by finding considerable diversity of clinical picture within the schizophrenia spectrum. They have not found evidence for a genetic component in acute forms of schizophrenia. Evidence for the causal role of psychosocial factors has been reported from some of these investigations.[15]

Genetic factors can be considered in terms of either static or dynamic neurobiological models and in terms of structural or functional bases for pathology. The gene(s) code protein synthesis, but consequences of altered synthesis may be functional and/or structural, and effects could be direct or could contribute to more complex disorganization of physiological and then psychosocial systems. In the past, the major focus of many genetically oriented investigative groups was the search for abnormal enzymes that could generate behavioral abnormalities. Currently, however, the most common focus is the search for altered enzymatic activity, such as in monoamine oxidase.

Biochemical Etiologies

The View from Pharmacologic Models

Biochemical etiologies of schizophrenia have been studied with particular success through the use of pharmacological models. It is interesting to note, however, that the original breakthroughs in psychiatric pharmacotherapeutics did not emerge from biochemical theories of disease, except in the case of lithium, where initial interest was based on an incorrect hypothesis. Rather, psychopharmacological innovations have been based primarily on clinical observations of unexpected pharmacological effects (e.g., the antidepressant effect of isoniazid in tuberculosis patients). Then, when drugs were noted to have effects on cognition, mood, or behavior, the study of their mode of action often led to biochemical hypotheses of mental illness. The catecholamine depletion hypothesis of depressive illness followed the introduction of catecholamine-depleting antidepressant medications, and the dopamine hypothesis in schizophrenia followed the introduction of dopamine-blocking drugs for the treatment of that disorder.

It is important to note this sequence of exploration, because it limits the use of treatment efficacy as a validating criterion for most biochemical hypotheses of psychiatric disorder. Fortunately, in these two instances (the catecholamine depletion hypothesis of depression and the dopamine hypothesis of schizophrenia), the biochemical theory of etiology has been further reinforced by a second set of pharmacological observations. Depressive episodes are associated with catecholamine-depleting drugs (e.g., reserpine) and psychotic symptoms can be induced by dopamine agonists (e.g., amphetamine). This confluence of pharmacological data strengthens the biochemical hypothesis but is still not definitive for demonstrating etiology. Pharmacological observations lead to attractive and potentially testable hypotheses of causation, but the crucial next step requires demonstrating not only that they can cause the disorder but that they actually are causative factors. Pharmacological agents may correct or exacerbate dysfunction without being or modifying a basic causal factor.

Drugs that influence cough suppression may or may not be closely related to the etiology of the cough.

In other ways as well, the pharmacological model has both important strengths and limitations. This model has given rise to an explosion of valuable new knowledge about brain physiology, and clinical studies with psychiatric patients promise advances in the scientific base of clinical practice. At the same time, this model has been difficult to use specifically for understanding schizophrenia, since all antipsychotic drugs developed so far are not highly discriminating, appearing to have therapeutic effects for all psychotic illnesses. More importantly, no drug yet available has a comprehensive treatment action in schizophrenia. Therapeutic value for some aspects of the syndrome is not necessarily accompanied by therapeutic efficacy for other aspects. We are best at psychotic symptom reduction and have little knowledge of pharmacotherapy for social impairment or intrapsychic deterioration. Clinicians may not agree on a definition of the "core" of schizophrenia, but few of us believe that any current therapeutic technique strikes at the heart of the disorder.

Methods for developing pharmacological treatments of schizophrenia also tend to limit the possible etiological implications these agents have regarding causality. Observing the behavioral effects of dopamine antagonists in laboratory animals has been the screening technique to test the antipsychotic activity of new drugs. This is a useful technique for new drug development, but its limitations for increasing the understanding of etiology should be readily apparent. Such a system can only produce dopamine-blocking antipsychotic drugs and does not have the potential for development of radically different pharmacological approaches to schizophrenia. The fact that most antipsychotic drugs occupy dopamine receptors does not provide overwhelming support for the dopamine theory, since only dopamine blockers pass the preclinical screening tests most commonly used for antipsychotic drugs.

Starting from another point, if a pharmacological substance could induce a reasonable simulation of schizophrenia, investigating the mode of action of this substance might be valuable for understanding etiology. Pursuing this line of reasoning, particular attention has been given to psychotomimetic drugs and amphetamine. In fact, the amphetamine psychosis is a most convincing human model in its mimicry of acute, good prognosis, paranoid schizophrenia. This effect, together with the dopamine-blocking action of antipsychotic drugs, gives increased support to the dopamine hypothesis of schizophrenia. However, while amphetamines and psychotomimetic drugs simulate some aspects of schizophrenia, they are limited in that they fail to induce the complex psychopathology (e.g., postpsychotic intrapsychic and interpersonal deterioration) often associated with the disorder.

The problem of a pharmacological approach to understanding etiology is further complicated by the implausibility of producing schizophrenia in animals. This roadblock severely limits the neurobiologist's capacity to investigate brain functioning which might be implicated as an etiological factor. Referring to a rigid rodent as catatonic and treating it as though a reasonable facsimile of the human phenomenon had been achieved shows how desperate we are for valid models of schizophrenia.

Two Current Chemical Hypotheses

The Dopamine Hypothesis. As we noted above, the dopamine hypothesis is the major biochemical theory of schizophrenia today. The dopamine hypothesis states that schizophrenia results from excessive transmission in dopaminergic neuronal pathways (presumably mesolimbic and/or mesocortical). The data supporting this hypothesis are pharmacological in nature. Antipsychotic drugs impede dopaminergic transmission while dopamine agonists (e.g., amphetamine) may provoke symptoms in patients and mimic some aspects of psychosis in nonpatients.[16-18] Although antipsychotic drugs have many biochemical actions, the role of dopaminergic blockade is emphasized because of the close correlation between the clinical potency of these drugs and their potency at the dopamine receptor. Antipsychotic drugs also affect other biogenic amine (e.g., noradrenergic) neurotransmitter systems, but the level of activity at dopamine neurons correlates most closely with clinical potency.[16-19]

The evolution and implications of the dopamine hypothesis reflect the strengths, limitations, and vigor of neurobiological research on the "functional" psychoses. The dopamine hypothesis, derived as it is from pharmacological evidence, is a particularly good working hypothesis for the mode of action of antipsychotic drugs. The fit between theory and fact is excellent in many regards. However, the dopamine hypothesis, even when applied only to antipsychotic drug action, has certain limitations. These are: (1) The main effect of antipsychotic drugs may be on neurotransmitters, modulators, or networks not yet identified; (2) the drugs have multiple actions in the brain, and therapeutic effect may be based on a combination, sequence, or balance of actions rather than on a single predominant effect; and (3) early and late effects on neuronal systems are different. Rapid behavioral effects associated with initial administration may reflect the drug's occupying postsynaptic dopamine receptors, hence reducing message transmission through these receptors. However, the system adjusts to this acute blockade, and therapeutic effects several weeks later may depend on reactive or adaptive physiological processes which neutralize the short-term pharmacological effects. The major complication of long-term antipsychotic medication, tardive dyskinesia, suggests such a sequence. Current hypotheses view tardive dyskinesia as a secondary consequence of the acute dopamine blockade, namely, reactive supersensitivity in dopamine neurons and/or cholinergic/dopaminergic imbalance. This is not the whole story, of course, but it is clear from this and longitudinal biochemical studies that acute and chronic drug exposure have different effects on dopamine neurons.

These considerations notwithstanding, the dopamine hypothesis of antipsychotic drug action has provided an excellent means of organizing neuropharmacological data. But its utility as an etiological hypothesis of schizophrenia is more open to question. On the positive side, dopamine agonists may sometimes worsen schizophrenia, and a dopamine-degrading enzyme, monoamine oxidase, is decreased in the platelets of some schizophrenics. But these findings do not prove that dopaminergic dysfunction is a cause of schizophrenia. The distinction between finding correlations and demonstrating actual cause–effect sequence must be recalled, and no such sequential chain has been proven.

Many investigators have even attempted to find direct evidence for heightened dopaminergic activity in schizophrenia, but to date none has been convincingly successful. These negative results have led some investigators to conclude that the dopamine hypothesis of schizophrenia can be rejected. That conclusion, however, is extreme. It fails to recognize that, at the current stage of psychiatry, experiments for proving or disproving any hypothesis definitively are rare indeed. In definitively exploring biological hypotheses of schizophrenia, it is probably essential, but usually impossible, for clinical scientists to have direct access to the relevant brain tissue in the living patient. Without such access, we cannot, for example, record directly from limbic neuronal projections to determine their firing rate or sample the biochemical processes of these cells. Adequate *in vivo* studies would provide the ideal solution, but such studies are often unethical or technically difficult to achieve.

The types of current problems with *in vivo* approaches can be readily illustrated. Attempts to assess increased turnover of brain dopamine assumed to occur during psychosis demonstrate several of the major problems. *In vivo* studies to identify such increased turnover have used cerebrospinal fluid as an accessible tissue in which to measure dopamine metabolites in schizophrenic patients. Excessive activity in the dopamine neurons may be reflected in more rapid synthesis and degradation of dopamine, and its metabolites (e.g., homovanilic acid) may accumulate more rapidly and in greater quantity than in normals. When this hypothesis was tested, most schizophrenic patients did not deviate from normal standards or from control subjects; hence, the hypothesis was rejected. However, the collectable cerebrospinal fluid may not have been adequate to reflect increased turnover in the key mesolimbic and mesocortical dopamine systems even if such turnover did exist. Of the dopamine metabolites in spinal fluid, 90% or more are derived, not from mesolimbic and mesocortical systems, but from the nigrostriatal pathways. Furthermore, if dopamine receptors were hypersensitive, the neurons might fire at an increased rate without increased neurotransmitter metabolism.

Other attempts at assessing the dopamine hypothesis also are plagued by problems with study paradigms unable to provide decisive results. For example, the study of neuroendocrine secretions (e.g., prolactin, growth hormone) in blood and urine may provide little information about neurophysiology critical to schizophrenia because so many regulatory mechanisms are involved in the secretion of these substances. Furthermore, inferences to schizophrenia from dopamine systems involved in neuroendocrine regulation are complicated since the neuroendocrine-regulating dopamine systems are not the systems implicated in schizophrenia and may not be analogous in their level of activity.

One method of studying the precise site of biochemical abnormality implicated in schizophrenia is by biochemical and histochemical investigations of the brains of schizophrenic patients collected at autopsy. This, of course, permits direct access to limbic system tissue. However, this approach is also replete with methodological and logistic problems. At the time of study, the complex integrated functions of the brain have ceased. Even if the biochemical composition (e.g., concentration of a neurotransmitter or activity of an enzyme) of an important locus such as the nucleus accumbens differs from comparison brains, one cannot judge whether the overall harmony of the integrated neural networks was disrupted during life. And, of course, there is the further problem that abnormalities in postmortem brain material from schizophrenic patients may derive from factors that accompany schizophrenia rather than cause it. Such factors include exposure to drugs, nutritional deficiencies, and other conditions to which schizophrenic patients are exposed that may lead to brain change.

A recent report[20] attracted attention by claiming to provide direct evidence for the dopamine theory of schizophrenia by finding an abnormally high number of dopamine receptors in the limbic regions. But neuroleptic medication may have induced this alteration, since it has been shown to increase the number of binding sites for dopamine at the synaptic cleft in laboratory animals. This problem might be controlled by studying postmortem brains of schizophrenics never exposed to drugs. Such a study is impractical, however, because most people who have been diagnosed as schizophrenic have received drug treatment and it is difficult to construct a valid diagnosis after death in persons never diagnosed as schizophrenic during their life. Sparse clinical data and lack of systematic diagnostic evaluation are often a particularly weak link in postmortem studies. Logistical problems involved in obtaining brains, minimizing time from death to autopsy, rapid extraction of brain from cranium and freezing of tissue, further hamper this method of inquiry.

Many of the problems with postmortem study could be circumvented if schizophrenic patients requiring neurosurgical procedures for other illnesses could be investigated. In such a possibility, a new set of complications comes into play, however. Artifact from anesthesia, preoperative stress, nonschizophrenic brain pathology, surgical trauma and many other practical and ethical concerns have made such studies (e.g., recording from depth electrodes) rare and, thus far, uninformative about the dopamine hypothesis.

To demonstrate the nature of the information base in exploring etiology, we have emphasized the problems in such research. Nevertheless, at this point we conclude that the dopamine theory of antipsychotic action is carefully formulated and extensively reinforced by experimental data and that it probably provides a partial explanation for why neuroleptic drugs reduce psychotic symptoms in schizophrenia and other psychotic disorders. Although we also conclude that the dopamine theory of schizophrenia has merit, it is speculative, devoid of direct experimental support, and only modestly supported by indirect evidence.

The nature of the evidence has been discussed at some length to clarify the two sides of an important coin. First, when data seem to affirm a biological hypothesis of schizophrenia, the meaning of this confirmation must be measured in relation to the study's capacity to assess the overall harmony and integration of the relevant brain systems. If the hypothesis is etiological, the design's capacity for separating cause and effect must be scrutinized. Second, when data fail to support a biological hypothesis, rejection of the hypothesis must be tempered against the inability of current research designs to provide decisive negative as well as positive results.

Understanding the neurobiology of schizophrenia will be achieved in piecemeal fashion, and solving the puzzle will require arranging and rearranging small pieces, discarding some and acquiring new ones. While some avenues of investigation may shed no light specifically on schizophrenia, many will contribute new knowledge and new concepts of brain physiology and of the brain/mind interface.

The Transmethylation Hypothesis of Schizophrenia. The transmethylation hypothesis[8,21] is another important biochemical hypothesis of schizophrenia etiology, one particularly valuable for illustrating the evolution of a biochemical model for schizophrenia. The long history of this hypothesis reflects the movement in the field of biological psychiatry during the past 25 years. The transmethylation hypothesis is distinguished from many biological hypotheses of schizophrenia in that it is derived neither from observations of schizophrenic patients nor from the study of the mode of action of drugs used in the treatment of schizophrenia. Rather, it is based on knowledge of brain metabolic pathways, the effect of psychedelic drugs on behavior, and the structural similarities between mind-altering chemicals and endogenous brain substances.

During the late 1940s, interest in a model of schizophrenia based on psychosis induced by exogenous compounds was growing. Several investigators and theoreticians proposed that hallucinogenic compounds produced model psychoses. It is now clear that psychotic states created by drugs such as mescaline, LSD, and DMT are imperfect models, involving only selected aspects of schizophrenia; but these earlier proposals provided valuable beginnings in a field devoid of suitable paradigms for studying this disorder.

Osmond and Smythies[22] noted that norepinephrine and mescaline were similar chemicals and realized that methylation of a norepinephrine phenolic (hydroxyl) chain would create a compound structurally similar to mescaline. It was later discovered that catabolism of dopamine and norepinephrine produced compounds of even greater structural similarity to mescaline and that there were notable similarities between endogenous indoles such as serotonin and hallucinogenic indoles such as LSD, DMT, and psilocybin. The transmethylation hypothesis was simple, to the point and, above all, testable, modifiable, and retestable. Perhaps naturally occurring neurotransmitter substances could be metabolically transformed into hallucinogenic (or schizophrenogenic) compounds providing a biochemical basis for the observed clinical phenomena.

Establishing the validity of biological hypotheses of schizophrenia proceeds in three steps: (1) demonstrating biological plausibility; (2) demonstrating a meaningful association with schizophrenia; and (3) providing evidence for causality. Using transmethylation to illustrate, the following conditions would establish plausibility: (a) the precursor biochemicals are present in humans; (b) a metabolic pathway for transmethylation exists in humans; (c) the methylated compounds are biologically active in humans, producing biological or psychological effects associated with schizophrenia and/or exacerbating biological and/or psychological manifestations in schizophrenic patients; (d) if an endogenous metabolic pathway is not plausible, then an exogenous source of the hallucinogenic substances must be identified.

The transmethylation hypothesis was established on the assumption that precursor substances were endogenously available. What needed to be demonstrated was that compounds identical to known hallucinogens are produced or that endogenous biochemicals have hallucinogenic properties.

The following data support the possibility of such a mechanism in humans. The human brain contains the enzyme required for methylating hydroxyl groups of catecholamines (O-methylation) and the enzyme required for N-methylation of indole amines. Methylated amines have been identified in humans. Some of these compounds (e.g., DMT, bufotenine) are definite or probable hallucinogenic substances. Thus, the brain research carried out between 1950 and 1975 has established a foundation for the possibility of the transmethylation hypothesis.

The gap between possibility and probability, however, has swallowed virtually every hypothesis put forward in schizophrenia, whether biological or psychosocial. The next step in the transmethylation inquiry was to find an actual association with schizophrenia. Demonstrating quantitative or qualitative differences between schizophrenic subjects and nonschizophrenic subjects on indices reflecting precursors, enzymatic activity, or methylated hallucinogenic amines was one approach used. Exploring whether schizophrenic and nonschizophrenic subjects responded differently to pharmacological manipulation of these metabolic processes was another approach. Such pharmacological probes could examine the consequences of changing precursor availability, increasing or decreasing methyl donors, altering enzymatic activity, or counteracting the effect of methylated hallucinogens with methyl acceptors. The pursuit of this evidence required clinical investigations that were, and still are, fraught with design difficulties such as drug and environmental artifact, subject selection, limitations on direct access to brain metabolic functioning, and nonspecificity of pharmacological manipulation.

With these problems in mind, we can summarize attempts to establish an association between the transmethylation hypothesis and schizophrenia. First, studies attempting to show that schizophrenic patients differ from other subjects quantitatively or qualitatively in supposed endogenous hallucinogenic compounds, precursors or metabolites of these compounds, or methylating enzymes have produced some promising findings.[8,21] However, difficulties replicating findings and controlling artifact, together with occasional convincing negative results (e.g., finding supposed hallucinogens in normal controls but showing neither uniqueness nor increased frequency in schizophrenic subjects),[23] resulted in only marginal direct support for the transmethylation hypothesis.

The history of the pink spot (dimethoxyphenylethylamine) is illustrative.[8] This transmethylated metabolite of dopamine was identified in the urine of schizophrenic subjects, but not in control groups. Further refinement and investigation showed quantitative, but not qualitative, differences between the two groups, and still further study suggested that those differences may have been artifacts of patient diet rather than concomitants of pathology.

Other studies have purported to find hallucinogenic metabolites in the urine of schizophrenics, but not in control subjects. However, when more rigorously controlled clinical investigations, including the study of patients off medications, were carried out, results failed to establish a difference between schizophrenic subjects and nonschizophrenic subjects in the level of previously implicated transmethylating enzyme activity or methylated biogenic amine metabolies.

A second strategy has involved producing schizophrenic exacerbation or schizophrenia-like symptomatology with methyl donors, or decreasing manifest symptomatology by reducing availability of methyl donors. A series of studies examining the effect of methyl donor loading consistently showed that symptom exacerbation can be achieved in schizophrenic patients.[8,21] This is the best evidence supporting the transmethylation hypothesis as relevant to schizophrenia, but even this evidence is open to alternate interpretations, such as viewing the clinical changes as nonspecific toxic effects. The most effective strategies for further exploration of this aspect of the hypothesis have involved using a monoamine oxidase inhibitor to reduce catabolism while administering substantial doses of the methyl donor methionine. Such strategies appear not to induce schizophrenia-like conditions in normal subjects but do produce an exacerbation among symptomatic schizophrenic patients.

Nicotinic acid and related compounds function as methyl acceptors. Should the transmethylation hypothesis be valid, administration of methyl acceptors might reduce the formation of transmethylated psychotogenic substances by competing for methyl groups. The clinical evaluation of this proposition was first carried out in 1952 by Hoffer and Osmond.[22] The initial results with nicotinic acid and nicotinamide adenine dinucleotide appeared promising, but a number of replication attempts have failed to provide affirmative evidence, and methyl acceptors failed to prevent or reverse psychotic exacerbation produced by methyl donors.[8,21,24] Furthermore, the administration of methyl acceptors has not been shown to affect the methylating process in normal metabolism.

There are severe limitations in the experimental designs of the above studies, and a definitive test of the transmethylation hypothesis is not yet possible. While equivocal results are confusing and negative results are discouraging, keep in mind once again how difficult it is to conduct human experiments which can produce definitive evidence in this area. Negative findings may result from an inability to select the proper subgroup of patients for study. Artifact can hide true positive cases as well as produce false positives. The biochemist may have inadequate techniques (e.g., assay insensitivity or instability) or be measuring the wrong biochemicals and enzymes. Metabolic pathways that initiate schizophrenic psychosis may be altered but no longer be abnormal at the time the subject is studied.

As we noted earlier, it is far easier to establish an association between a biological variable and schizophrenia than it is to demonstrate a causative role for that variable. Most studies are conducted on patients during psychotic episodes without the longitudinal design that could clarify sequential relations, let alone cause and effect. Since psychotic states are associated with many psychobiological changes, these changes should be considered concomitants rather than causes of the psychotic process until proven otherwise. Finding an elevation of stress-sensitive hormones during psychotic states would hardly incriminate endocrine factors as etiological!

Summarizing the status of the transmethylation hypothesis, some studies report quantitative and/or qualitative differences in transmethylated compounds found in schizophrenic patients and their relatives. There is evidence that methyl donors worsen schizophrenic symptoms and a suggestion that methyl acceptors provide therapeutic relief. In spite of such supporting data, however, the weight of evidence fails to confirm the transmethylation hypothesis. While transmethylating enzymes and precursor biochemicals are found in humans, no difference in transmethylating enzyme activity is reported in schizophrenic subjects. The more effectively controlled studies are less successful in distinguishing schizophrenic from other patient and control subjects in biochemical assessment of transmethylated compounds. Therapeutic response to methyl acceptors such as nicotinic acid has proved difficult to replicate. Methionine loading, especially if given with enzyme inhibitors, consistently exacerbates symptomatology in schizophrenics, but it is not clear that this methyl donor effect is a distinguishing feature of schizophrenia, since patients with other psychoses have not been adequately studied.

Other Related Biological Hypotheses Briefly Noted

Among the many relevant biological hypotheses of schizophrenia etiology that exist, we have focused on some major genetic and biochemical hypotheses to illustrate concepts, findings, methods, and limitations in the study of the clinical biology of schizophrenia. The reviews listed at the end of the chapter give more detailed information on these and other biological hypotheses regarding schizophrenia. We have omitted the studies of neuromuscular dysfunction,[21,25] although these investigations are important for their consistency and replicability and for demonstrating both enzymatic (creatine phosphokinase) and morphological changes associated with psychotic states. The findings of these studies are particularly fascinating because they were not predicted by any of the major theories of schizophrenia. On the other hand, interest is dampened by the fact that these factors do not clearly distinguish schizophrenic patients from those with affective disorders, and also because it is difficult to know or to demonstrate what the relationship between the biological findings and the clinical picture might be.

The demonstration of a *slow virus* etiology for several perplexing neurological disorders (e.g., kuru, Jakob–Creutzfeldt disease) has renewed interest in viral theories of schizophrenia.[26] Long the domain of a few Soviet scientists, viral hypotheses have received recent impetus from descriptions of schizophrenia-like psychoses associated with viral illness, documentation by epidemiologists that late winter births are more frequent in schizophrenia (perinatal viral exposure being one possible explanation), and occasional reports of laboratory findings consistent with viral infections in schizophrenic patients (e.g., increases in cerebrospinal fluid or serum immunoglobulin factions, higher viral antibody levels, binding viral particles in cerebrospinal fluid). However, of those studies completed to date, positive findings are inconsistent and apply only to a minority of patients. Control standards are not always available to assure that findings actually deviate from the norm or are unique to schizophrenia, and all known neural illnesses with established viral etiology have confirming morphological changes. This last fact does not disaffirm a viral hypothesis for schizophrenia, since the histopathology of limbic systems of schizophrenic patients has not been exhaustively studied; but skepticism is warranted.

Some of the protein findings supporting the viral inquiry (i.e., immunoglobulins) are also compatible with immune and autoimmune hypotheses.[27] There is fairly consistent data to indicate acute phase serum protein reaction in schizophrenia, but this occurs in other psychiatric disorders and trauma and is not specific to schizophrenia. Work reported in the Soviet literature and investigations by Frohman and his colleagues[28] continue to raise the possibility of pathognomonic deviations in protein (the α_2-globulin or so-called S protein, for example). Heath's pioneering and controversial work attempting to demonstrate a pathogenic autoimmune phenomenon has been discounted because of some failures in replicating and difficulties in reproducing the human experiments. Heath's protein appears to be a gamma globulin, and he offers extensive evidence from serum studies and postmortem brain studies to support an autoimmune theory.[29] Autoimmune hypotheses have been pursued with negative or inconsistent findings by other workers. As with viral models, it must be emphasized that schizophrenia does not appear to be analogous to known autoimmune diseases (e.g., characteristic tissue lesions, systemic symptoms, enlarged thymus, therapeutic response to corticosteroids, and genetic association with other autoimmune diseases).

Considerable attention has been given to the role of *enzymes* in the biochemistry of schizophrenia. The research on monoamine oxidase (MAO) is one particularly important focus of such efforts. MAO is an attractive enzyme in regard to schizophrenia etiology, since it is involved in the metabolism of biogenic amines, its activity in platelets is (to some extent) a heritable trait, and it is readily available in peripheral tissues for assay. Observing less MAO activity in platelets of chronic schizophrenic patients than in other psychiatric patients or normal subjects led Murphy, Wyatt, and others to associate this enzyme tentatively with schizophrenia.[30] Finding similar low levels of activity in monozygotic twins discordant for schizophrenia raised the possibility that MAO was a genetic marker for vulnerability to schizophrenia.[31] MAO studies would be supportive of the dopamine hypothesis of schizophrenia or for the importance of other potentially pathogenic amines such as phenylethylamine.

The initial reports from Murphy and Wyatt have been subjected to many replication attempts, some affirming and others refuting[30]. There appear to be substantial patient subgroup differences in platelet MAO activity, with chronic schizophrenic patients having less enzyme activity than normals or patients with acute schizophrenia[32] (chronic alcoholics and patients with affective disorder being intermediate).[30] However, it is uncertain whether platelet MAO reflects brain MAO activity; and in initial examination of postmortem brain tissue, MAO activity failed to discriminate schizophrenic patients from other subjects.

Despite the significant group differences in MAO activity, overlap is extensive; MAO levels, therefore, are not presently useful as a diagnostic tool. This is similar to other biological findings, such as eye-tracking dysfunction reported by Holzman and others,[33] in which group differences are established but overlap between groups limits the usefulness of the measure as an assessment of individual psychopathology. It should be noted, however, that the pattern of some replications and some failures is what would be expected if a finding were valid for some homogeneous subgroup of a heterogeneous population. A constant challenge in schizophrenia research is to define these subgroups rather than to reject possibly valid hypotheses prematurely.

We have not touched on orthomolecular theories beyond mentioning the role of nicotinamide as a methyl acceptor. To date, this provocative area has been associated more with advocacy than with scientific verification. Diagnostic and treatment procedures have been zealously promulgated without the critical caution which seems advisable to most clinical scientists. Some defenders of the theory have posited that organized psychiatry finds the basic tenets of orthomolecular psychiatry repugnant. On the contrary, biological psychiatry has a time-honored interest in the transmethylation hypothesis, an interest in the effects of nutrients (i.e., precursor amines) on brain physiology, the psychopathological implications of deficiency states, and the potential that trace minerals and neurotransmitter precursors (e.g., choline) may have for therapeutic impact even in nondeficiency states. Mainstream psychiatry's failure to embrace the orthomolecular movement is not based on an innate disregard for all of its concepts, but rather on a negative assessment of evidence to date and an innate disregard for ideologically based "science." Excellent reviews and commentary are available.[34-36]

Psychophysiology and Schizophrenia

Psychophysiology has as its domain the measurement of nervous system electrical activity or its consequences on effector systems (e.g.; voluntary musculature, sweat glands, respiration). The psychophysiological approach is used to study physiological systems in relationship to biological and psychological states and behavioral patterns.[37,38] This field of science, together with the study of perception, attention, and cognition,[39-41] bridges the gap between biochemistry and clinical observation. The psychopathology hypotheses of psychophysiologists are intuitively understood by clinicians and require only brief mention here. Not so well understood are the precise definitions and variables used and the nature of inferences to be drawn from psychophysiological data.

Psychophysiological topics of relevance to schizophrenia include such concepts as arousal, information processing, attention, response sets, and habituation. The concept of altered arousal, for example, appears to be of immediate relevance to the clinician when he observes patients who are withdrawn and silent and exhibit motor retardation, or who are pressured and agitated and experience sleep disturbances. Information-processing and other concepts which focus on inability to select stimuli, maintain attention, or prevent stimulus overload as the bases of psychopathology seem validated when one attempts to understand what, why, and how a psychotic patient is communicating.

While the concepts of psychophysiology are appealing, the multiplicity of variables and the complexity of methods and interpretations have caused many clinicians to remain unfamiliar with the scientific base and promise of this discipline. For example, the clinical EEG would have been a welcome ancillary diagnostic tool had conventional recordings been informative for individual cases of schizophrenia. At times useful in confirming or excluding other disorders, the clinical EEG has appeared to have no specific role for diagnosing or understanding schizophrenia. However, special techniques employing computer technology have resulted in a dazzling array of investigative tools and potentially valuable findings. Power spectrum analysis has affirmed group differences (e.g., schizophrenics have weak alpha, heightened beta, and increased delta activities), and patients with very stable records may be less responsive to antipsychotic drug treatment.[42] Computer techniques[43-46] for averaging EEG records permit assessment of specific brain electrical responses to discrete stimuli. Precise timing allows examination of early, middle, and late components of such "evoked" potentials, and components which arise from different anatomic locations reflect different stages and aspects of information-processing. Some of these research procedures do not require that the patient pay attention to a particular stimulus or problem. Thus, this approach to investigating information processing has a decided advantage in the study of profoundly disturbed patients for whom the problem of active cooperation had been a recurrent impasse to psychological research.

Processes of arousal[37,47] were an early focus in psychophysiology. Is our withdrawn, mute patient attempting to reduce stimulation to his overaroused nervous system? Does his behavior reflect a state of hypoarousal? A pulse or blood pressure determination might answer this question (if our patient happens to be a cardiovascular responder). Activity of the sweat glands may be informative if our patient is responsive in this system. Limbic system involvement makes various attributes of skin conductance further springboards for theorizing and research. Some workers have observed pupil size to be increased in schizophrenic patients with a reduction in size following neuroleptic administration. Pupil size is controlled by parasympathetic and sympathetic input and is influenced by limbic structures, external events (e.g., bright light), attention, and information processing. Should we focus our attention on this complex organ?

There is obviously a multitude of complicated approaches toward even this one psychophysiological concept, arousal. The field is difficult to follow and comprehend for several other important reasons as well:

1. Many of the variables are state phenomena, and test results vary over time and have many artifacts.

2. Various measures purported to reflect a single concept (e.g., arousal) may have low correlations with each other; hence, heart rate may be fast, respiration slow, and skin conductance normal in the same patient. This makes conceptualization and research extremely difficult with even the most basic concepts.

3. Schizophrenic subjects tend to span the normal range on most psychophysiological measures but are often characterized by greater heterogeneity (or skew toward both extremes) than do control populations. This is an important finding but will be confusing to the investigator and bewildering to the casual observer until criteria for defining more homogeneous patient subgroups are devised.

4. To date, the most interesting findings are based on group differences, and prospective studies which may determine the value of psychophysiological assessment in the individual patient (or high risk subject) are in their early stages.

Despite the many complications, psychophysiological studies are an extremely promising, perhaps crucial, part of the attempt to understand the etiology of schizophrenia. These studies have the potential of bridging the biochemical–clinical gap by providing explanations of how genetic/biochemical factors are expressed in behavior. Generally, they involve safe, relatively available techniques that provide the most direct and objective measures reflecting integrated brain functioning in intact human subjects. The immediacy of a specific brain wave response to a given stimulus contrasts with the peripheral and static nature of assaying a dopamine metabolite in cerebrospinal fluid which has accumulated over an undetermined time from many neural tissues. When psychophysiological data are collected concurrently with biochemical data, their combined power may even help pinpoint anatomic loci of dysfunction or drug action.

The field of psychophysiology is further enhanced by the rapidly developing technologies for investigating the basic physiology of the human brain. For example, regional xenon-131 blood flow studies have been carried out with chronic schizophrenic patients showing that they have low frontal and high posterior blood flow. It has been possible to "spot" small areas of increased metabolism (i.e., blood flow) associated with hallucinations, speech, thought without action, etc.[50]

Taking still another direction of potential value, some leading psychophysiologists have investigated vulnerability to schizophrenia utilizing paradigms assuming that psychophysiological variables such as abnormalities in stimulus management may reflect a predisposition to schizophrenia. Such a predisposition is seen as proceeding through other steps that determine the chain of events that leads to psychopathology. Since some psychophysiological variables are highly heritable, this research approach links directly to genetic studies and may be useful for marking risk populations.[37,47–49]

Now that we have sketched these general directions and potentialities of psychophysiological research on the etiology of schizophrenia, a more detailed illustration of one current paradigm will be useful. Skin conductance orienting response (SCOR) has received considerable attention during the past 10 years following primate research by Bagshaw and others showing that amygdalectomy produced low SC and hippocampectomy produced hyperresponsivity on SC measures. Limbic structures were known to be susceptible to hypoxic damage, and Mednick and Schulsinger had reported an increase in perinatal complications in the children they studied who were at high risk for schizophrenia.[49]

Pursuing direct evaluation of a possible relationship between SC and schizophrenia, Venables and his co-workers[48] noted that up to half of adult schizophrenics were non-SCOR responders, compared to normal controls, whose nonresponse rate was less than 10%. Of the schizophrenic subjects who did respond, many failed to habituate and thus could be considered hyperresponders. Thus, schizophrenic subjects in these experiments tended to be at both extremes of response disposition.

Since these earlier studies, many components of the SCOR have been examined among subjects who are responders. The time required for a stimulated response to recover to baseline has been of special interest, since a fast recovery of SC has been shown to characterize high risk children who later developed psychopathological states.

Some investigators such as Zahn[47] have failed to replicate certain earlier results, e.g., to find an impressive bimodal distribution of schizophrenic subjects into nonresponders and hyperresponders. Although such studies have cast doubts on a possible etiological role of SC in schizophrenia, the many positive findings are impressive to many workers, including Zahn.

The complexity of the phenomena involved may well account at least in part for the conflicting results obtained. One illustration of this complexity is a statement by Zahn summarizing data on two autonomic patterns and various genetic and environmental precursors that may contribute to schizophrenia:

> If one accepts the results of these studies at face value, a possible conclusion is that autonomic hyper-responsivity to sensory stimulation and slow habituation are accompaniments of being at high risk for schizophrenia that are determined by genetic factors (or by interactions of genetics with early environmental variables such as pregnancy and birth complications) and that high tonic arousal found in high risk subjects is determined by a pathologic childhood environment.[47]

In studies of the psychophysiology of schizophrenia, as with the genetic and biochemical research, it is outside the task of this book to review or even illustrate the full range of work being accomplished. We will close this discussion, however, by noting that several psychophysiological areas of immediate relevance to clinical care are being explored. To cite only a few: Itil[42] has shown an association between EEG patterns and responsiveness to antipsychotic drugs; Monroe[51] has demonstrated that activated EEG procedures are useful in discriminating between schizophrenia and an acute episodic "third psychosis"; Buchsbaum and colleagues[52] have discriminated good prognosis from poor prognosis schizophrenia with average evoked response EEG measures and have found that combining evoked response and a biochemical variable (platelet MAO) was more effective than either alone in diagnostic discrimination[53]; and Zahn and colleagues,[54] using a prospective design, have shown that autonomic nervous system variables had a predictive relationship to short-term outcome in drug-free acute schizophrenic patients. Good, comprehensive reviews of these efforts are listed at the end of this chapter.

A FEW CAVEATS

Kety's[55,56] 1959 critique of biological methods had a salutary effect on the field, and methodological rigor has increased. In general, investigators now refine their methods to control for conspicuous artifact and acknowledge uncontrolled factors. However, certain principles are still important in evaluating biological research on schizophrenia. One must be wary of any investigation where the reliability of techniques used to assess biochemical, psychological, and clinical variables has not been demonstrated in the investigator's laboratory. Where possible, validity should also be evaluated. The clinician unfamiliar with the tools of basic science should realize that techniques in biology are often imprecise and subject to interpretation. It is tempting to assume that investigator bias will not affect "objective" assay data, but there is much room for subjective interpretation in both the qualitative and quantitative aspects of substance identification. One scientist's specificity is another's contaminated peak!

The heterogeneity of schizophrenic populations plagues all investigators studying more than one patient. Since we do not have the definitive clinical tools to identify homogeneous illness groups, it follows that even the biological investigator whose theory is valid may be able to confirm his hypothesis in only a subgroup of his subjects. Refutation from replication attempts may be based on the inability to select similar subjects in subsequent studies. Even replication failures by the original contributor may be based on an inability to recognize the critical variables in subject selection. Failures to replicate challenge the original results but often are themselves not definitive.

The clinician who daily attempts to make sense of complex psychopathology will appreciate the investigator's inability to identify homogeneous subgroups on descriptive grounds. When a biological hypothesis is tested in 10 patients and confirmed in only 2, we must conclude that the hypothesis was not confirmed. However, the 2 exceptions may be taken seriously, and the investigator is justified in further attempts to define the relevant subpopulation. Too often, valuable leads are discarded because we assume schizophrenic patients to be a single entity, and "outliers" are ignored.

Another problem, one noted earlier as well, is that the distinctively human nature of schizophrenia may preclude any satisfactory animal model of the disease(s). This fact has a profound effect on the rate at which new knowledge can be acquired. The existing models (e.g., amphetamine, LSD, amygdalectomy) do not provide the research leverage to the schizophrenologist that cultured cancer cells give to the oncologist.

It should also be recognized that current neurotransmitter hypotheses are restricted to those biochemicals now known to regulate and transmit messages in the brain. New neurotransmitters and neuroregulators are being identified at a rapid pace (more than 30 such biochemicals are now known). There is excitement about these new developments, but it should also remind us that at present we have insufficient knowledge of brain physiology to be certain that our hypotheses deal with the most crucial biochemicals, neuronal tracts, or reciprocal and interacting neuronal systems.

Hypotheses in any field of science should lend themselves to falsification. Often enough, hypotheses relevant to schizophrenia are not subject to crisp affirmation or disaffirmation. With biological hypotheses, evidence required to confirm or reject an hypothesis, at least, can be imagined. As we noted above, it has been difficult to subject these hypotheses to definitive tests because of the inadequacies of clinical, biochemical, and physiological techniques and the inaccessibility of implicated brain areas for *in vivo* study. Frustration is inevitable, but many biological hypotheses have, at the very least, spawned work generally informative concerning brain functioning. Neurotransmitter hypotheses have led to greater understanding of neurophysiology and neuroanatomy, despite their limited contribution to understanding psychiatric illness.

The human brain is a wonderfully complex and adaptive organ system. The many mechanisms of compensation for or adaptation to altered physiology in some component may obscure abnormalities and mislead the investigator. If there were a genetically induced increase in the biosynthesis of dopamine in neurons terminating in the nucleus accumbens, we would expect local compensation such as increased inhibitory feedback in GABA pathways, decreased receptor sensitivity, and increased activity of catabolizing enzymes. When one considers the tens of thousands of synaptic connections relaying information more distally, the coping possibilities seem endless. Study paradigms informative about each of these systems may suggest different views of schizophrenia (e.g., hypergabaminergic disease). Pieces of the puzzle accumulate, but a better understanding of the overall harmony of brain physiology will be required before the meaning of isolated functional deviance can be understood.

A final problem is that the limbic system, assumed to be critical in the neurophysiology of schizophrenia, is also the presumed substrate for stress and distress and, together with neocortical brainstem, hypothalamic structures, and the pituitary gland, plays a central role in adaptation. This is a wonderful arrangement for human functioning, but it confounds investigation of schizophrenia. To have a stress-sensitive organ as the object of study under stressful circumstances is a methodological nightmare, unless stress itself is the scientific focus. When it seems that we are studying schizophrenia, we may be studying simply the psychobiology of stress. When we fail to confirm a biological hypothesis, such as dopamine hyperactivity in schizophrenic patients, we may be recording the biology of adaptation. This is one reason for giving special emphasis to the study of subjects at high risk for schizophrenia who have not yet decompensated, or to the study of recovered subjects no longer in clinical distress. Such designs may minimize the effects of clinical state, although adaptation processes may still obscure findings or confound interpretation.

THE NEW BIOLOGISTS OF SCHIZOPHRENIA

Earlier in this chapter, we described the lack of esteem for biological psychiatry held by the mainstream of American psychiatry during the middle third of this century. This was based in part on the intense interest in, and dedication to, psychological constructs for explaining psychiatric disorders. But it was also based on the oversimplification by the biologically oriented of clinical phenomena into biological constructs, coupled with immodest claims for the explanatory or therapeutic power of new ideas and findings. Impressive findings were all too often later explained by artifact or simply found unreplicable by other laboratories—fuel for the polemic fires!

The situation today is quite different, in part because of the serendipitous discovery of psychotherapeutic drugs. Establishing the efficacy of neuroleptic medication for psychotic states and of antidepressant medications for depressive disorders demanded that psychiatry attend to the brain side of the brain–mind dialectic. This boost to biological psychiatry was balanced by the fact that these important discoveries were not the result of new biological theory, but rather were fortuitous clinical observations.

New tools and incentives for biological investigation have been forthcoming, and the biological psychiatrist is now armed with more complex neurobiological concepts, more definitive and replicable neurochemical techniques, more respect for the perplexing psychological and biological heterogeneity of psychiatric illnesses, more knowledge of animal behavioral neurochemistry, and a more critical perspective in reporting the work accomplished. Although the rise of biological psychiatry came about in part for the wrong reasons, it was timely and well deserved.

How far the field has come can be illustrated most graphically by one final example, the opiate receptor story.[57-59] The simple possibility that synthesized pharmaceuticals which directly affect brain physiology might have endogenously occurring counterparts had long been neglected. In 1973, several groups identified the opiate receptor, and efforts to identify naturally occurring substances active at this site rapidly bore fruit. Endorphins are endogenous substances which act as neuroregulators at the opiate receptor. The identification of several endorphins (e.g., two pentapeptides, leucine and methionine enkephalins) and the clarification of their structural relationship to larger peptide hormones (e.g., beta-lipotropin, ACTH) have opened the door to discovery of a new brain system with previously unknown neuropathways, neurotransmitters, and neuromodulators. Twenty years ago, such a discovery might quickly have been linked with schizophrenia, and sweeping etiological and/or therapeutic claims would have been expected. However, this time the difficult work of hypothesis testing and model building is generally proceeding in advance of attempts to reorient psychiatry.

The neuroanatomists and histochemists have noted that neuroactive peptides localize in specific pathways, some of which are concentrated in brain areas associated with mood regulation. Neuropharmacological behavioral studies have demonstrated a range of behavioral responses to opioid peptides; some of these responses were morphine-like, and some were similar to the effects of other psychoactive drugs. The relatively high concentration of enkephalins in limbic structures increased the interest of the behavioral neurochemist, and the demonstration of a cataleptic effect with the administration of endorphins suggested a pharmacological animal model for one aspect of behavioral disturbances associated with schizophrenia. This new information was used to supplement previous clinical observations of behavioral changes in drug addicts. Earlier reports speculated that opiate use was a form of self-medication for mental disturbance. Opiates were reported to be tranquilizing, to overcome feelings of inadequacy, and to reduce paranoid ideation and pathological regression. More recent experience suggests that narcotic-addicted schizophrenic patients benefit from methadone maintenance.

Based on this type of information, tentative hypotheses have been suggested concerning the possible role of endorphins in mental illnesses such as schizophrenia. Initial hypotheses must be simplistic, considering present limitations of information. Some evidence suggests that the schizophrenic patient may have a relative deficiency of physiological functioning in opiate receptor systems, while other evidence supports a hypothesis of relative hyperactivity of these systems. To date, a few clinical studies have been done which test these hypotheses. Terenius *et al.*[60] have identified substances in the cerebrospinal fluid of psychiatric patients which have the chemical activity of methionine–enkephalin. These substances were found in several patients diagnosed as schizophrenic, manic, or depressed, with decreasing amounts found on clinical recovery. In an open trial with naloxone (opiate antagonist) hallucinated schizophrenic patients showed remarkable reduction in hallucinatory behavior.[61] The indecisiveness of an open trial was readily appreciated, and several replication attempts using double-blind methodology (one by the original investigators) failed to show a therapeutic effect of naloxone.[62-65] Dose and patient selection, of course, are critical factors in such investigations, particularly when rapidly metabolized pharmacological substances are involved. Further investigations with higher doses of naloxone (or the longer-acting naltrexone) are more promising[66] but still inconclusive.

An alternate hypothesis, that endorphins may be therapeutic rather than causative in schizophrenia, has not yet been carefully evaluated. Kline *et al.*[67] administered beta-endorphins to a number of psychiatric patients in an open design and reported impressive improvement in most patients without regard to diagnostic category. This report was greeted with skepticism within biological psychiatry. While these investigators stated the need for replication in controlled studies, the field had grown intolerant of claims emerging from preliminary investigations, even when accompanied by cautionary notes. Recently, a double-blind placebo-controlled study of β-endorphin reported statistically significant but clinically trivial changes in schizophrenic subjects.[68]

The endorphin story is just beginning to be written. The description above is intended to convey something of the promise and rigor that often are currently associated with neurobiological and clinical investigations related to the brain physiology of psychotic conditions. At present, no definite structural or functional brain abnormality has been satisfactorily implicated in the etiology and pathogenesis of schizophrenia, but the field of biological psychiatry has matured. It is presently armed with sophisticated concepts, new clinical methods, and new technology in behavioral biochemistry and physiology. With these developments, there is every promise of important and rapid advances in understanding the human brain in both normal and disordered function.

SUMMARY

Great progress has been made in studying biological aspects of schizophrenia. Improved methods and more cautious claims of success have combined to further the exploration of several leads regarding possible biological etiologies. The evidence for a genetic contribution is now compelling, indeed, but the modes of action for genetic factors and their applicability to all forms of schizophrenia remain uncertain. None of the major biochemical and psychophysiological factors—abnormalities in dopamine metabolism, transmethylation, endorphins or autonomic response—have been definitively demonstrated as etiologic, but available evidence suggests the possibility of such etiologic factors and points the way to further study. As the roles of these and other biologic contributions become clearer, we believe that they will best be understood as part of a broader interactive etiologic model that also includes psychological and social factors.

RECOMMENDED READING

Freedman, D. X. *Biology of the major psychoses: A comparative analysis.* New York: Raven Press, 1975.

Kety, S. S. Biochemical theories of schizophrenia. A two-part critical review of current theories and of the evidence used to support them. *Science*, 1959, 129:1528–1532, 1590–1596.

Kety, S. S. Current biochemical approaches to schizophrenia. *New England Journal of Medicine*, 1967, 276:325–331.

Schizophrenia Bulletin, 1976, 2(1).

Schizophrenia Bulletin, 1977, 3(1).

Snyder, S. H., Banerjee, S. P., Yamamura, H. I., and Greenberg, D. Drugs, neurotransmitters, and schizophrenia. *Science*, 1974, 184:1243–1253.

Spohn, H. E., and Patterson, T. Recent studies of psychophysiology in schizophrenia. *Schizophrenia Bulletin*, 1979, 5(4):581–611.

Stevens, J. R. An anatomy of schizophrenia? *Archives of General Psychiatry*, 1973, 29:177–189.

Wyatt, R. J., Termini, B. A., and Davis, J. Biochemical and sleep studies of schizophrenia: A review of the literature—1960–1970. Part 1. Biochemical studies. *Schizophrenia Bulletin*, Fall 1971, 1 (Experimental issue 4):10–44.

REFERENCES

1. Freud, S. A project for a scientific psychology. In: *The standard edition of the complete psychological works of Sigmund Freud*, Strachey, J. (ed.). London: Hogarth Press, 1966, 1:283–398.

2. Searles, H. F. *Collected Papers on Schizophrenia and Related Subjects*. New York: International Universities Press, 1965.

3. Wynne, L. C., Singer, M. T., Bartko, J. J., and Toohey, M. L. Schizophrenics and their families: Recent research on parental communication. In: *Developments in psychiatric research*, Tanner, J. M. (ed.). London: Hodden & Stoughton, 1977, 254–286.

4. Bleuler, E. *Dementia praecox*. New York: International Universities Press, 1950.

5. Freud, S. On narcissism: An introduction, 1914. In: *The standard edition of the complete works of Sigmund Freud*, Strachey, J., and Freud, A. (eds.). London: Hogarth Press, 1957, 14:67–102.

6. Weinberger, D. R., Bigelow, L. B., Kleinman, J. E., Klein, S. T., Rosenblatt, J. E., and Wyatt, R. J. Cerebral ventricular enlargement in chronic schizophrenia. *Archives of General Psychiatry*, 1980, 37:11–13.

7. Kleinman, J. E., Bridge, P., Kavorem, F., Speciale, S., Staub, R., Lalcman, S., Gillin, J. C., and Wyatt, R. J. Catecholamines and metabolism in the brain of psychotics and normals: Postmortem studies. In: *Catecholamines: Basic and clinical frontiers*, Usdin, E., Kopin, I. J. and Barchas, J. D. (eds.). New York: Pergamon Press, 1979, 1845–1847.

8. Wyatt, R. J., Lermini, B. A., and Davis, J. Biochemical and sleep studies of schizophrenia: A review of the literature, 1960–1970: Part 1. Biochemical studies. *Schizophrenia Bulletin*, 1971, 4, 10–44.

9. Selye, H. Stress and the general adaptation syndrome. *British Medical Journal*, 1950, 2:1383–1392.

10. Arlow, J. A., and Brenner, C. *Psychoanalytic Concepts and the Structural Theory.* New York: International Universities Press, 1964.
11. Matthysse, S. W., and Kidd, K. K. Estimating the genetic contribution to schizophrenia. *American Journal of Psychiatry*, 1976, 133:185–191.
12. Rieder, R. O., and Gershon, E. S. Genetic strategies in biological psychiatry. *Archives of General Psychiatry*, 1978, 35:866–873.
13. Gottesman, I. I., and Shields, J. A critical review of recent adoption, twin, and family studies of schizophrenia: Behavioral genetics perspectives. *Schizophrenia Bulletin*, 1976, 2:360–401.
14. Kety, S. S., Rosenthal D., Wender, P. H., and Schulsinger, F. The types and prevalence of mental illness in the biological and adoptive families of adopted schizophrenics. In: *The Transmission of Schizophrenia*, Rosenthal, D., and Kety, S. S. (eds.). Oxford: Pergamon Press, 1968, 345–362.
15. Wynne, L. C., Singer, M. T., and Toohey, M. L. Communication of the adoptive parents of schizophrenics. In: *Schizophrenia 75: Psychotherapy, family studies, research*, Jorstad, J., and Ugelstad, E. (eds.). Oslo: Universitetsforlaget, 1976, 413–452.
16. Janowsky, D. S. and Davis, J. M. Dopamine, psychomotor stimulants, and schizophrenia: Effects of methylphenidate and the stereoisomers of amphetamine in schizophrenia. In: *Neuropsychopharmacology of Monoamines and Their Regulatory Enzymes*, Usdin, E. (ed.). New York: Raven Press, 1973, 317–23.
17. Janowsky, D. S., El-Yousef, M. K., Davis, J. M., and Sekerke, H. J. Provocation of schizophrenic symptoms by intravenous administration of methylphenidate. *Archives of General Psychiatry*, 1973, 28:185–191.
18. Snyder, S. H., Banerjee, S. P., Yamamura, H. I., and Greenberg, D. Drugs, neurotransmitters, and schizophrenia. *Science*, 1974, 184:1243–1253.
19. Seeman, P., Lee, T., Chau-wong, M., and Wong, K. Antipsychotic drugs, doses and neuroleptic/dopamine receptors. *Nature*, 1976, 261:717–718.
20. Lee, T., Seeman, P., Tourtellotte, W. W., Farley, I. J., and Hornykeiwicz, O. Binding of ^{3}H-neuroleptics and ^{3}H-apomorphine in schizophrenic brains. *Nature*, 1978, 274:897–900.
21. Rosengarten, H., and Friedhoff, A. J. A review of recent studies of the biosynthesis and excretion of hallucinogens formed by methylation of neurotransmitters or related substances. *Schizophrenia Bulletin*, 1976, 2:90–105.
22. Osmond, H., and Smythies, J. Schizophrenia: A new approach. *Journal of Mental Sciences*, 1952, 98:309–315.
23. Carpenter, W. T., Fink, E. B., Narasimhachari, N., and Himwich, H. E.: A test of the transmethylation hypotheses in acute schizophrenic patients. *American Journal of Psychiatry*, 1975, 132:1067–1071.
24. McGrath, S. D., O'Brien, P. F., Power, P. J., and Shea, J. D. Nicotinamide treatment of schizophrenia. *Schizophrenia Bulletin*, 1972, 5:74–76.
25. Meltzer, H. Y. Neuromuscular dysfunction in schizophrenia. *Schizophrenia Bulletin*, 1976, 2:106–135.
26. Torrey, E. F., and Peterson, M. R. The viral hypothesis of schizophrenia. *Schizophrenia Bulletin*, 1976, 2:136–146.

27. Durell, J., and Archer, E. G. Plasma proteins in schizophrenia: A review. *Schizophrenia Bulletin*, 1976, 2:147–160.
28. Frohman, C. E., Harmison, C. R., Arthur, R. E., and Gottlieb, J. S. Conformation of a unique plasma protein in schizophrenia. *Biological Psychiatry*, 1971, 3:113–121.
29. Heath, R. G. An antibrain globulin in schizophrenia. In: *Biochemistry, Schizophrenias and Affective Illness*, Himwich, H. E. (ed.). Baltimore: Williams & Wilkins, 1971, 171–197.
30. Wyatt, R. J., Potkin, S. G., and Murphy, D. L. Platelet monoamine oxidase activity in schizophrenia: A review of the data. *American Journal of Psychiatry*, 1979, 136:377–385.
31. Wyatt, R. J., Murphy, D. L., Belmaker, R., Cohen, S., Donnelly, C. H., and Pollin, W. Reduced monoamine oxidase in platelets: A possible genetic marker for vulnerability to schizophrenia. *Science*, 1973, 179:916–918.
32. Carpenter, W. T., Jr., Murphy, D. L., and Wyatt, R. J. Platelet monoamine oxidase activity in acute schizophrenia. *American Journal of Psychiatry*, 1975, 132:438–441.
33. Holzman, P. S., and Levy, D. L. Smooth pursuit eye movements and functional psychoses: A review. *Schizophrenia Bulletin*, 1977, 3:15–27.
34. Ban, T. A., and Lehmann, H. E. Nicotinic acid in the treatment of schizophrenia. Part 2. *Canadian Psychiatric Association Journal*, 1975, 20:103–112.
35. Leff, D. N. Megavitamins and mental disease. *Medical World News*, August 11, 1975, 71–82.
36. *Task Force Report 7: Megavitamin and orthomolecular therapy in psychiatry.* Washington, D.C.: American Psychiatric Association, 1973.
37. Spohn, H. E., and Patterson, T. Recent studies of psychophysiology in schizophrenia. *Schizophrenia Bulletin*, 1979, 5:581–611.
38. Buchsbaum, M. S. Psychophysiology and schizophrenia. *Schizophrenia Bulletin*, 1977, 3:7–14.
39. Chapman, L. J. Recent advances in the study of schizophrenic cognition. *Schizophrenia Bulletin*, 1979, 5:568–580.
40. Garmezy, N. The psychology and psychopathology of attention. *Schizophrenia Bulletin*, 1977, 3:360–369.
41. Matthysse, S. The biology of attention. *Schizophrenia Bulletin*, 1977, 3:370–372.
42. Itil, T. M. Qualitative and quantitative EEG findings in schizophrenia. *Schizophrenia Bulletin*, 1977, 3:61–79.
43. Callaway, E., Tueting, P., and Koslow, S. *Event-related potentials in man.* New York: Academic Press, 1978.
44. Buchsbaum, M. S. The middle evoked response components and schizophrenia. *Schizophrenia Bulletin*, 1977, 3:93–104.
45. Roth, W. T. Late event-related potentials and psychopathology. *Schizophrenia Bulletin*, 1977, 3:105–120.
46. Shagass, C. Early evoked potentials. *Schizophrenia Bulletin*, 1977, 3:80–92.
47. Zahn, T. P. Autonomic nervous system characteristics possibly related to a genetic predisposition to schizophrenia. *Schizophrenia Bulletin*, 1977, 3:49–60.
48. Venables, P. H. The electrodermal physiology of schizophrenics and children

at risk for schizophrenia: Controversies and developments. *Schizophrenia Bulletin*, 1977, 3:28–47.

49. Mednick, S. A., and Schulsinger, F. Some premorbid characteristics related to breakdown in children with schizophrenic mothers. In: *The Transmission of Schizophrenia*, Rosenthal, D., and Kety, S. S. (eds.). New York: Pergamon Press, Ltd., 1968, 267–291.

50. Franzen, G., and Ingvar, D. H. Abnormal distribution of cerebral activity in chronic schizophrenia. *Journal of Psychiatric Research*, 1975, 12:199–214.

51. Monroe, R. R. *Eposodic Behavioral Disorders: A Psychodynamic and Neurophysiologic Analysis*. Cambridge: Harvard University Press, 1970.

52. Landau, S. G., Buchsbaum, M. S., Carpenter, W. T., Strauss, J. S., and Sacks, M. Schizophrenia and stimulus intensity control. *Archives of General Psychiatry*, 1975, 32:1239–1245.

53. Coursey, R. D., Buchsbaum, M. S., and Murphy, D. L. Psychological characteristics of subjects identified by platelet MAO activity and evoked potentials as biologically at risk for psychopathology. *Journal of Abnormal Psychology*, 1980, 89:151–164.

54. Zahn, T. P., Carpenter, W. T., Jr., and McGlashan, T. H. Autonomic nervous system activity in acute schizophrenia. II. Relationships to short term prognosis and clinical state. *Archives of General Psychiatry*, in press.

55. Kety, S. S. Biochemical theories of schizophrenia. Part I. *Science*, 1959a, 129:1528–1532.

56. Kety, S. S. Biochemical theories of schizophrenia. Part II. *Science*, 1959b, 129:1590–1596.

57. Watson, S. J., Akil, H., Berger, P. A., et al. Some observations on the opiate peptides and schizophrenia. *Archives of General Psychiatry*, 1979, 36:220–223.

58. Snyder, S. H. The opiate receptor and morphine-like peptides in the brain. *American Journal of Psychiatry*, 1978, 135:645–652.

59. Vereby, K., Volavka, J., and Clouet, D. Endorphins in psychiatry. *Archives of General Psychiatry*, 1978, 35:877–888.

60. Terenius, L., Wahlstrom, A., Lindstrom, L., and Widerlov, E. Increased CSF levels of endorphins in chronic psychosis. *Neuroscience Letters*, 1976, 3:157–162.

61. Gunne, L. M., Lundstrom, L., and Terenius, L. Naloxone-induced reversal of schizophrenic hallucinations. *Journal of Neural Transmission*, 1977, 40:13–19.

62. Davis, G. C., Bunney, W. E., DeFraites, E. G., Kleinman, J. E., Van Kammen, D. P., Post, R. M., and Wyatt, R. J. Intravenous naloxone administration in schizophrenia and affective illness. *Science*, 1977, 197:74–77.

63. Janowsky, D. S., Segal, D. S., Bloom, F., Abrams, A., and Guillemin, R. Lack of effect of naloxone on schizophrenic symptoms. *American Journal of Psychiatry*, 1977, 134:926–927.

64. Kurland, A. A., McCabe, O. L., Hanlon, T. H., and Sullivan, D. The treatment of perceptual disturbances in schizophrenia with naloxone hydrochloride. *American Journal of Psychiatry*, 1977, 134:1408–1410.

65. Volavka, J., Mallya, A., Baig, S., and Perez-Cruet, J. Naloxone in chronic schizophrenia. *Science*, 1977, 196:1227–1228.

66. Watson, S. J., Berger, P. A., Akil, H., Mills, J. J., and Barchas, J. D. Effects of

naloxone on schizophrenia: Reduction in hallucinations in a subpopulation of subjects. *Science*, 1978, 201:73–76.

67. Kline, N. S., Li, C. H., Lehmann, H. E., Lajtha, A., Laski, E., and Cooper, T. Beta-endorphin-induced changes in schizophrenic and depressed patients. *Archives of General Psychiatry*, 1977, 34:111–113.

68. Berger, P. A., Watson, S. J., Akil, H., Elliott, G. R., Rubin, R. T., Pfefferbaum, A., Davis, K. L., Barchas, J. D., and Li, C. H. β-endorphin and schizophrenia. *Archives of General Psychiatry*, 1980, 37:635–640.

CHAPTER 8

Etiologies of Schizophrenia

PSYCHOLOGICAL AND SOCIAL

The interactive developmental model described in Chapter 2 involves psychological and social factors as well as biochemical, psychophysiological, and genetic characteristics. All are necessary for an integrated concept of schizophrenia. This chapter will focus on the four major types of psychosocial characteristics for which there is appreciable evidence of etiological importance in schizophrenia: early psychosocial development, family characteristics, the broader social environment, and stressful life events.

The recommended readings at the end of this chapter include detailed works aimed at elucidating one or another specific psychosocial area of pathogenic significance. It is important to appreciate in reading such works that investigators of complex phenomena often control or even ignore (hopefully only for a limited time) many important aspects of the phenomena in order to study in depth those variables they judge of greatest interest. This occurs with the neurobiologist as with the psychoanalyst. It is our hope, nevertheless, that the reader of those references, perhaps with some help from this book, will be able to see past a particular proponent's orientation and independently integrate salient features into a broader model of psychopathology.

EARLY PSYCHOLOGICAL DEVELOPMENT

Just as there are several paradigms for considering biological causes of schizophrenia, so there are various approaches to considering psychosocial etiologies. As is so often true in science, the assumptions and hypotheses of each paradigm are closely interwoven with a particular research or clinical method providing the "window" through which the theory is developed.

One major orientation to the etiology of schizophrenia is the developmental approach. As might be expected, this approach is most often used by those who have worked with children, seen given patients over extended periods of time, or otherwise focused on developmental perspectives or methods likely to produce developmental data. Without necessarily denying genetic and constitutional factors, these students of schizophrenia conceptualize vulnerability to the disease as psychological characteristics developed progressively in childhood.

It is important, and perhaps surprising, to note that many psychiatrists and other mental health professionals do not assume that factors in psychological development are important to the genesis of schizophrenia. From their viewpoint, schizophrenia is seen as an innate biological condition activated in adolescence or later, with symptoms possibly triggered by stress of some kind. One must keep this alternative orientation in mind while considering developmental theories and data.

Much of the research on developmental etiologies of schizophrenia has been retrospective. This often allows considerable bias and leaves key variables uncontrolled. To overcome these problems, one of today's most promising study paradigms has been implemented in a number of centers—namely, the prospective study of children at high risk for schizophrenia. In such studies, the selection criteria for children usually require that they be the offspring of a schizophrenic mother, hence increasing risk tenfold. This is true from an epidemiological perspective, but of course it is not yet clear how much this increased risk is genetic and how much is environmental. Other strategies for defining groups at risk utilize environmental or psychophysiological criteria, such as family disruption and unusual physiological response patterns, or even study subjects already disturbed in adolescence but not yet with diagnosable schizophrenia.

Most of these risk studies are still in early and midphase, and more definitive results must await the passage of the subject children through young adulthood to determine which actually develop schizophrenia. However, in a recent review of risk research, Chapman[1] noted frequent findings of reaction time deficits to standard stimuli in children of schizophrenics, increased errors in attentional functioning as measured in the continuous performance test, and also cognitive defects similar to those seen in adult schizophrenics. The other variables investigated in these prospective studies reach well beyond cognitive functioning to include a wide range of biological, psychological, and social factors that may reflect increasing vulnerability to schizophrenia as the children pass through developmental phases.

The risk study findings, as they accumulate, should provide much valuable information directly, but they may also clarify the mechanisms of several abnormalities already documented by another vast literature, the studies of premorbid adjustment.[2] These studies have been particularly notable for their many replications and unusually high degree of validity. They have documented many important psychosocial development characteristics as precursors to schizophrenic disorders. It has been found, for example, that certain types of behavior in school-age children–passivity in girls and passivity or aggressiveness in boys–predict the increased likelihood of schizophrenia at a later age.[3] Several of these studies have used school and other records written prior to illness in order to minimize retrospective falsification and bias. A large number of premorbid adjustment studies have also documented that certain developmental processes such as poor "premorbid" social relations and work function preceding schizophrenia influence the course of illness, but it remains a moot point whether such factors are best conceptualized as premorbid and pathogenic or early morbid and indicative of already established illness.

Beyond such systematically collected data suggesting important psychological precursors to schizophrenia, there is a considerable body of theory based on clinical observations also providing evidence that early life stages involve patterns of psychological functioning contributing to the occurrence of schizophrenia at later stages. Psychoanalytic and psychodynamic hypotheses have been prominent in this regard. Among these, deficit theory and conflict theory are two particularly important orientations.[4]

Deficit theory states that individuals who become schizophrenic have some kind of lack that is a precursor to the disorder. The basic deficit is sometimes regarded as constitutional and not explorable in psychological terms, yet contributing to psychological deficit, for example, by impeding object relationships with the mother and others. Or the early deficit (for example, in relating) may be seen as arising directly from early life experiences of deprivations.

In either case, subsequent failures in cognitive and affective development may be viewed as direct reflections of the deficit, perhaps as generating, and evidenced by, progressively impaired psychosexual development. The child reaches each new developmental task less well prepared and less capable of accomplishing that task, even within a favorable psychosocial context. Coping mechanisms may permit the child to develop, albeit falteringly, within a protective familial environment, but at some point (often when the person is challenged to establish an independent life) such brittle adjustment collapses and psychotic decompensation follows.

Conflict theory provides a second view of possible preschizophrenic development. It is based on the assumption that certain intrapsychic conflicts are pathogenic. This view often conceptualizes the conflict as beginning at the earliest developmental levels.[5,6]

Some conflict theories are based on observations of certain types of interactions between the infant and its closest relations (especially the mother), which are assumed to generate psychological defenses in the child that make it vulnerable to schizophrenia. The defenses may, for example, protect against rage toward a withdrawn mother or may represent projective identification with pathological components of the father. The psychological mechanisms for defense against intense feelings and impulses distort reality—projection and denial are examples—laying the groundwork for psychotic symptoms later in life.

A third major view of possible early psychological characteristics that predispose to schizophrenia is derived from concepts of maladaptive learning. Although several learning (including behavioral) theories have been suggested,[7] one has, in the past at least, been particularly influential. That is the view of Adolph Meyer,[8] who suggested that schizophrenia may involve increasingly abnormal behaviors learned over time. Possibly, through chains of reward and/or punishment, slightly abnormal responses to stimuli may evolve as increasingly abnormal, becoming fixed and dominating the person's life. As with other developmental orientations, this view neither assumes nor denies innate factors. However, it emphasizes learning and experience while deemphasizing the contributions of unconscious processes and fantasy. Such a theory can readily incorporate biological factors, since damaged circuitry in reward centers or habituation processes could serve as original contributors to distorted development.[9]

The various developmental orientations to the question, "How does a person come to be vulnerable to schizophrenia?" are not mutually exclusive. Deficit, conflict, and maladaptive learning might occur in many combinations. We must, however, await more specific data to validate any of the theories and demonstrate the precise connections between psychosocial development and schizophrenia. It seems inconceivable, however, that understanding vulnerability to schizophrenia can be accomplished without at least some understanding of behavioral, intrapsychic, and social aspects of the individual's developmental history.

Besides the potential of research in this area for discovering more about vulnerability, it may also help us acquire new information about paths to other unusual outcomes, such as creativity.[10] The extent to which various classes of illness have distinct rather than common development may also be clarified.

Studies of psychosocial and neurobiological development promise information crucial to the prevention of schizophrenia, since the developmental factors which produce vulnerability can also yield information for reducing it. And, of course, the fact that there are genetic and constitutional factors in some (or all) forms of schizophrenia does not reduce one whit the potential for prevention at a variety of points along the way before it becomes manifest.

FAMILY FACTORS

Mapping the distribution of illness in families has been an effective strategy for confirming the existence of genetic factors in schizophrenia, but this approach to "family studies" is not the only one. In fact, the genetic family study paradigms have not been suited to test environmental theories except those that assume that the presence of an ill relative leads to the same illness. In this regard, pedigree and adoptive studies have not supported the existence of family environment etiologies of schizophrenia, but family theorists have rarely suggested that living with a psychotic relative is a crucial variable in the etiology of schizophrenic disorders. This, of course, does not deny other profound implications of living with or being reared by a psychotic person, but it emphasizes that family studies aimed at discovering family psychosocial etiologies have a different focus from most genetic research.

The major hypothesis of most family–environment studies of schizophrenia etiology is that patterns of communication and relating within family systems (not necessarily associated with already diagnosed schizophrenia in a parent) are thought to contribute to a member's becoming schizophrenic. Investigators pursuing this orientation believe that, since the family forms the basic environment of the developing child, family power structures, views of reality, and means of communicating help to establish the child's patterns of thinking, perceiving, and feeling. Family problems in any of these areas, therefore, might severely and adversely affect cognitive and affective development.

Originally, the conceptualization of dementia praecox as a disease entity tended to focus attention on the ill individual rather than on the social unit. Perhaps this orientation has prevented most clinicians and investigators from even being exposed to experiences that would provide a broader perspective on etiology. And yet, considering the profound effects of inter-animal trauma that have been demonstrated in young rats, dogs, and monkeys, and the extensive literature on clinical experiences with interpersonal trauma in young humans, it is surprising that family interaction only recently has become a specific and legitimate focus in considering the etiology of schizophrenia. Some of the earlier studies of dementia praecox did note, perhaps defensively, that patients developing this disorder came from "good families," suggesting that there was no disgraceful taint. Some investigators remarked, however, that people from families with a schizophrenic member sometimes did seem strange.

For whatever reason, a family interaction paradigm for schizophrenia was not considered seriously until 1948, when Freida Fromm-Reichmann[11] first published her theory of the schizophrenogenic mother, an attempt to define specific relationships between the behavior of one family member and the occurrence of schizophrenia in another. Fromm-Reichmann observed that mothers of schizophrenics were often cold and distant. She believed that the child's need for a warm, affectionate relationship had not been met and that this lack impeded the development of necessary psychological and social skills and created a susceptibility to schizophrenia.

The concept of the schizophrenogenic mother, in spite of its historical importance, has been weakened by the test of time. There are several reasons for this. First, subsequent experience showed the supposed pathogenic characteristics to be absent in many mothers of schizophrenics, and "schizophrenogenic" traits were noted in parents raising children who did not become schizophrenic. Second, characteristics put forward as schizophrenogenic by Fromm-Reichmann and others were not sufficiently defined to permit empirical testing, and no research paradigms for establishing cause and effect were available. Finally, the concept was too often applied clinically in a provocative, derogatory way, causing more alienation than understanding.

It is clear that the "schizophrenogenic mother" as originally conceptualized is neither a necessary nor universal antecedent to schizophrenia. On the other hand, the concept has not been demonstrated to be totally incorrect, and many clinical observers continue to believe that, at least for some children who later become schizophrenic, lack of warmth in the early family environment may be a contributing factor to later illness.

Other hypotheses about family interactions that may be etiological for schizophrenia have followed from the work of Fromm-Reichmann. In one important series of writings, Lidz et al.[12] expounded the view that family schism and skew were etiological contributors to schizophrenia. On the basis of intensive studies of a few families, these investigators suggested that severe splits between parents, or one parent's being especially dominant and the other submissive, were etiologically important. They observed the constellation of extremely submissive father and dominant mother to be especially likely to cause schizophrenia in male offspring, a theory actually not too distant from the schizophrenogenic mother concept of Fromm-Reichmann.

While some investigators studied intrafamilial power relationships and psychodynamics, others described patterns of intrafamilial communication that might affect the developing cognitive, perceptual, and affective mechanisms of the child. Bateson et al.[13] postulated the double bind as one such communication pattern. This concept involves a parent (or parents) communicating contradictory but imperative messages to the child. The child must resolve the mutually exclusive demands but cannot escape this paradox by leaving or clarifying it. Contradictory messages abound in life, of course, such as that of the mother who gives her son two ties and, seeing him wearing one, says, "What's the matter, don't you like the other?" More typical of a pathological double bind is the situation in which a child attempts to kiss his mother, who unconsciously withdraws and then says, "Why don't you kiss me?" When this type of interaction dominates relationships in an intense and troubled family where close relationships without hostility are viewed as essential, one can imagine the impact on the child's development.

It has been extremely difficult to test the double bind theory empirically, and a recent conference on this topic resulted in only partial success at developing the concept further.[14] The problem of whether the double bind is specific to schizophrenia, the question of the child's psychopathology leading to (rather than being caused by) such ambivalent modes of relating, and the issue of establishing reliable and valid methods for evaluating the occurrence of double bind have thus far proven difficult to overcome. Nonetheless, the double bind concept can be useful in organizing clinical observations and may still prove of etiological significance in subgroups of schizophrenic patients.

The communication theory that has been developed and tested with the most sophisticated research scrutiny is Wynne and Singer's concept of communication deviance.[15] These investigators demonstrated that parents of schizophrenics had several distinctive communication patterns that statistically differentiated them from parents of children with other psychiatric disorders or with no psychiatric disorder. The communication deviances included such characteristics as failure to arrive at closure, premature closure, and "lack of visualizability." It was hypothesized that children raised in an environment where these communication deviances dominated would have a compromised ability to deal conceptually with certain life demands.

Most of the research supporting this theory was carried out using parental couple responses to Rorschach tests. For this purpose, test protocols were not subjected to the standard methods usually employed for Rorschach interpretation but rather served as a sample of parental communication for specially designed scoring procedures. In developing this theory and research approach, Singer and Wynne have replicated and extended their original findings, as have other investigators. Data from sources other than the Rorschach have also been used.[16]

However, this work has recently been critically reviewed by Hirsch and Leff[17] in the context of a major replication attempt. These investigators also found that communication deviance statistically distinguished parents of schizophrenics from nonschizophrenics, but they reported a much less powerful discrimination than that found by Wynne and Singer. When quantity of words was controlled, the discrimination was lost, leading to a negative interpretation of the replication attempt results.

Wynne and colleagues argue that verbosity is a communication variable which may add to confusion. Reanalyzing their own data, however, they found that verbosity did not account for their findings, and other investigators[18] have since criticized the Hirsh–Leff use of statistical procedures that led to the apparent disconfirmation.

It will not surprise the reader of this book if we note here that the endeavor to understand the etiology of schizophrenia does not move forward in a simple linear fashion, any more than do quests in other areas of science. In our opinion, the Hirsh and Leff data may best be interpreted as suggesting less of an etiological role for parental communication deviance than the original findings, but not as refuting them. The differences may be due to methodological issues or may have arisen from sample differences generated by use of different diagnostic criteria. The Leff–Hirsh patients appear to have been diagnosed using a Schneiderian symptom, cross-sectional approach rather than focusing more on chronic or process characteristics, the kind more common in the sample of Wynne and Singer.

Another major approach to the possibility that family behavior contributes to the etiology of schizophrenia is the view that some families operate in a way that mystifies the child, isolating it from dealing with many aspects of the environment.[19] Wynne,[20] for example, described this view in noting the psychological "rubber fence" that surrounds certain families. Such a family isolates itself from others in a flexible yet impermeable way, keeping members closely tied to each other and away from outsiders. This theory also includes the view that perhaps some types of communication among family members exist, such as special "pseudomutual" communication, that appear to reflect agreement when little is present and help to generate and maintain this "rubber fence."

Pursuing further the hypothesis of special family communication patterns in schizophrenia using a methodologically rigorous experimental problem-solving design, Reiss found evidence to support an advanced version of the rubber fence, pseudomutual conceptualization. From a series of studies, he defined a typology of families, suggesting that families of schizophrenics were "consensus sensitive," that is, extremely sensitive to reaching agreement among themselves regardless of other aspects of reality, including objective task situations.[21]

The confluence of Reiss's laboratory data, the clinical and projective data of Wynne and his colleagues, and the observations of many clinicians who observe families is impressive indeed. This work has progressed further than most research dealing with possible specific family etiologies of schizophrenia, but since studies have been carried out in families where a member is already schizophrenic, cause-and-effect relationships remain elusive. The current vulnerability research mentioned earlier in this chapter may help to untie this knot.

Finally, another family environment characteristic potentially relevant to etiology comes from research on prognosis. Focusing on the impact of the family on schizophrenia outcome, a series of studies in London has revealed an astonishing impact of certain family communications on the course of the disorder. Because of the power of the findings, they also demand consideration as indicating a potential variable in etiology. Brown,[22] and then Vaughn and Leff,[23] have reported that high levels of "expressed emotion" (actually hostility and intrusiveness inferred from interviews with relatives) in the patient's family are associated with high rates of psychotic relapse, while low levels of "expressed emotion" may protect the vulnerable patient from relapse. This family variable appears to have an even more potent effect on relapse than drug maintenance. Expressed emotion is not a simple concept, however, and for further information Leff's review of this work is recommended.[24]

THE INTERACTIVE DEVELOPMENT MODEL

It is important to place views of the family environment as etiologically important in schizophrenia within the context of the interactive developmental model described in Chapter 2. To do so, take as a hypothetical case an infant born genetically vulnerable to schizophrenia. This genotype may be expressed as a nervous system vulnerable to hyperarousal and stimulus-overload. The infant may withdraw adaptively from stimulation, frustrating the mother's affectionate and caretaking activities. The mother may be very sensitive to rejection, or cool and aloof, perhaps protecting her system from overstimulation, having shared the same genotypic vulnerability.

Patterns of communication in the family unwittingly may have evolved to reduce stimulation, but this may be at the expense of full information sharing and potential for affective–cognitive integration. Conceptual confusion may ensue without apparent dysfunctional consequence, however, so long as the family unit is secure. But when the vulnerable adolescent attempts to deal with the expectation that he will leave home for college, the threat to the structural integrity of the family strains the system. Inability to reach a decision (or to clarify the essential considerations) fuels arguments that increase the affect and vindictiveness in the household.

The soon-to-be patient attempts his move. He lacks the interpersonal skills to reconstruct his environmental supports at college, finds the meaning and intent of communication confusing without the idiosyncratic parental clarifications, finds his psychological coping mechanisms overwhelmed (reducing anxiety with delusional interpretations based on denial and projection), and finds his hyperaroused nervous system overstimulated and decompensating.

In such a hypothetical and perhaps oversimplified scenario, one can see how difficult it is to reconstruct sequential relations, let alone tease out single causes and effects. By the same token, we hope it is clear that discarding such complex hypotheses because of the difficulty in providing definitive proof is silly pseudoscience. The psychosis that finally emerges is as likely to be fully explained by "faulty wiring" as the content of the evening news is to be explained by the wiring of a television set.*

CAVEATS

Having argued the validities of a family etiological impact on schizophrenia, we must now state a few caveats regarding theory and research.

1. We find no basis for explaining schizophrenia exclusively from a family point of view. Too many other important factors have been implicated as well. Besides, the fact that one child may be affected while others are not lends itself to no uniform explanation based on current family etiological theories alone. Each instance can be hypothesized away (e.g., specific vulnerability of the child, child born at a particular family stage, or the child reminding parents of a particular relative), but the conclusion is the same—no simple theory that family type X creates schizophrenic children is adequate. If family relationship patterns are etiological, they must interact with other factors, such as genetic or other biological variables or other environmental factors to produce schizophrenia.

2. Methods of study are unusually difficult since subtle, often unconscious patterns in a multiperson system are under investigation.

---

*With apologies to Paul MacLean[25] for paraphrasing his comments on thinking that the brain could account for human experience.

Beware of studies which seem to refute these concepts by using relatively simple approaches. For example, failure to find schizophrenia in adoptive parents of schizophrenic persons does not test any prominent family environment theory of schizophrenia.

3. As with most other nongenetic variables, cause and effect cannot be disentangled in ordinary clinical study designs. Prospective studies which begin data collection well in advance of manifest psychopathology in the offspring are crucial. The high risk design is the only practical approach to date.

4. In the last chapter we noted that a number of neurobiological hypotheses had generated new information about brain physiology even though they had not been validated as explanations of mental illness. Similarly, our knowledge of the human family has been enriched by the theories and observations described above, even though their value as etiological hypotheses of schizophrenia may remain in question.

5. It is difficult to underestimate the impact of a schizophrenic patient on his or her family. Burdens are great, emotions are powerful, and the mystery and social stigma of schizophrenia create special intrafamilial reaction patterns. Such patterns include denial, family isolation, rejection of the patient, and many other similarly negative responses.[26] One can see how readily these patterns could be interpreted in retrospect as inducing pathological change in the patient rather than as the family's reaction to pathological change in one of its members.

6. In spite of the methodological problems and limitations in data that continue to trouble the field, repeated findings indicate, as Riskin and Faunce[27] suggest, that certain basic variables in family communication are related to schizophrenia in offspring. These factors are (1) lack of clarity of speech, more often found in families with schizophrenic members; (2) failure to acknowledge or make a commitment to a response, as in overtly or covertly ignoring what others say and failing to make a clear definite statement of one's own; and (3) lack of humor, sometimes found in family members of schizophrenics.

THE SOCIAL ENVIRONMENT: LABELING, SOCIAL CLASS, AND CULTURAL PATTERNS

In no other area relevant to understanding schizophrenia is the ratio of fact to intensely held opinion so low. Beliefs abound that society induces schizophrenia in individuals or prevents it and even that schizophrenia itself is a cultural myth. For such important issues as these, socially sanctioned expertise often is no prerequisite for voicing "authoritative" opinions.

Many students of schizophrenia tend to ignore this problem, either because polemics discourage serious attention or because the relationship between the macroenvironment of culture and the single patient seems too abstract. However, interesting and informative observations and concepts relevant to the major questions are to be found, as well as some very solid and provocative data. The following discussions of labeling (societal reaction theory), social class, and culture may clarify the relevance of sociologic data to a medical model (interactive developmental) of schizophrenia.

Societal Reaction Theory and Labeling

Societal reaction and labeling theories state that societal reactions to individuals contribute to, or even cause, schizophrenia. Perhaps, it is believed, the ostracizing, isolating, or labeling effects of certain societal responses, such as considering someone "crazy" or "schizy," actually lead to the deviations imputed. The question raised in evaluating these theories of schizophrenia is how great and how specific the impact of a societal reaction is.

Social systems react to deviant individuals. This appears to be true for all species that live in groups. Do some forms of behavior which human society labels *deviant* (but which are not inherently schizophrenic) stimulate social responses which lead to further deviant behavior? This appears to be irrefutable. Numerous studies as well as clinical experience suggest the destructive impact of such reactions from the community on the vulnerable individual.[28,29]

Can such societal responses generate specifically diagnosable schizophrenic behaviors in vulnerable, or slightly deviant, individuals? If so, these societal responses should be sufficiently powerful and stereotyped to create specific behavioral abnormalities (schizophrenia), not just nonspecific abnormalities, such as generally increased deviance. Here the evidence is shaky, indeed.[30]

The step toward pure labelling theory is the question of whether some societal responses are capable of causing schizophrenia *de novo* in the previously nondeviant and/or nonvulnerable individual. If the answer to this question is yes, then a freestanding (nonillness) sociological model is tenable. If the answer is no, then societal reaction fits neatly into a developmental interactive model. In that case, it is a fairly direct extension of interpersonal and family theories of pathogenesis to include broader social factors.

We answer this last question in the negative. We find no compelling evidence to support a theory that societal reaction causes schizophrenia in an individual not already vulnerable or deviant. This may reflect our bias toward a broad medical model but seems the wiser position, considering the absence of decisive data affirming a pure sociological model. Furthermore, good evidence for genetic, gestational, perinatal, season of birth, and family environment contributions to etiology seems to preclude a narrow sociological position.

Yet, from our viewpoint, labeling is an important variable affecting the course, and perhaps the onset, of schizophrenia. The gross aspects of labeling are obvious to all. Who can doubt the devastating impact on a fragile person of perceiving that the entire social milieu regards him (wittingly or not) as subhuman, incurable, unmotivated, or incompetent to pursue ordinary expectations? What are the consequences on recovery in a society that determines that expensive health care from highly qualified specialists is not to be provided to the majority of patients with a certain illness? Can we doubt that a deteriorating course of disorder is fostered when fundamental roles are changed by social stigma and employment opportunities become limited?

But even the clinician who accepts such principles may be unlikely to acknowledge the profound effects of subtle reactions to which he is a party. For example, when schizophrenia is presumed, treatment decisions are often routinized rather than individualized. Rosenhan[28] recently, and Caudill[29] and Goffman[30] earlier, as well as many patients writing autobiographical accounts, have described a myriad of effects from professional care that may negatively affect the course of illness.

Our experience is that patients labeled "schizophrenic" are not victims of the treatment system. They come to doctors and hospitals seeking help for their suffering, and they receive far more help than harm. Schizophrenic withdrawal or other manifestations probably cannot be entirely explained by the aversive reactions of professionals involved with the patient, but the degree to which societal reactions to the ill person impact on his life is profound, and too many clinicians, administrators, and investigators avoid the empathy and introspection required to be cognizant of this aspect of pathogenesis.

In our view, the essence of the labeling process is the series of social reactions involving professionals as well as family, friends, employers, and the community more generally. ("Fans" used to sit in the stands and shout names like "Nut" and "Schizo" at Jimmy Pearsall, the Boston Red Sox outfielder who had been hospitalized for psychiatric disorder.) These reactions, heightened by the frightening and often unpredictable aspects of schizophrenia itself and the failure of professionals to work in sufficient depth with the patient's social context, complicate the patient's life, promote chronic disability, hinder recovery from this disorder, and may contribute to the origin of schizophrenia in the vulnerable person.

Cultural Factors

Speculations have been made that schizophrenia is the product of industrial cultures, of crowded living conditions, or of cultural systems with a particular pace or rigidity of life. In the past, cross-cultural differences in diagnostic practice, culturally determined response to inquiry, and shortcomings in epidemiological methods and sampling techniques have compromised studies of these questions and hindered the resolution of many issues regarding cultural factors in schizophrenia. However, in recent years, the development of operational diagnostic criteria, standardized approaches to collecting diagnostic information, and improved sampling methods for epidemiological study have provided answers to certain questions. For example, using a generally acceptable group of symptoms and signs as diagnostic criteria, schizophrenia has been found in every culture where it has been sought, and cases are remarkably similar in sign and symptom manifestations.[31,32] Incidence and prevalence data are more difficult to compare, but available data suggest surprisingly similar lifetime prevalence (about 1%) in diverse cultures. Some apparent exceptions[33] (e.g., Ireland, some areas of Africa) require further study to validate and explain the findings. On the whole, however, studies fail to support hypotheses that specific cultural factors are etiological for schizophrenia.

However, culture may be relevant to specific content and course of illness, if not to the incidence and occurrence of schizophrenia more generally. It is obvious (based on self-reports) that impulses, body movements, and thoughts are more likely to be caused by CIA-controlled computer-generated laser communications in Americans than in rural New Guineans. Similarly, the behavioral and affective concomitants of schizophrenia are also considerably influenced by cultural norms.[34]

Of more profound importance is the data now being reported suggesting that schizophrenia may run a more benign course in developing countries than in highly industrialized cultures.[35] These findings (if replicated) are clearly consistent with a theory that socioenvironmental factors influence the course rather than the onset of illness, but they may provide helpful leads to etiological factors as well. What the specific socioenvironmental characteristics might be that influence the course remains to be determined. But even before that is done, several important methodological issues in these findings need to be resolved. Alternate interpretations of the cultural differences found in course-of-schizophrenia data include the possibility that they are merely sampling artifacts. Schizophrenic patients who are less floridly psychotic and hence have a worse prognosis may not come for treatment (and therefore may not be available for study) in less highly developed countries. The possibility of a social explanation for better outcome in developing countries is made plausible, however, by postulating that schizophrenic patients in the countries in question (Nigeria, Colombia, India) are more likely to have available alternative social niches in their families, jobs, and communities than similar patients in more technologically developed countries.

The studies described above show that progress has been made in understanding cultural impact on schizophrenia and that certain myths have been dispelled. A theory of total cultural relativism or specificity can be ruled out, and even specific cultural determinants of schizophrenia risk appear to be minimal or rare. However, cultural impacts on the manifestations and course of disorder may be significant, and more specific information on these can provide a basis for focused exploration of cultural impact on etiology as well.

Social Class

One of the most frequently replicated findings in schizophrenia research is the higher concentration of schizophrenia in the lower social classes, a phenomenon especially marked in urban settings. But these findings do not necessarily indicate that the circumstances of lower class life are causal in schizophrenia. A noncausal view, the "downward drift" hypothesis, also explains some of the increased density of schizophrenia in the lower classes. Many schizophrenic patients "drift" down the social class ladder from their own earlier status or the status of their parents because of impaired role performance in school and occupation. It is these two characteristics, education and occupation, of course, that are generally used as measures of social class.

The work of Clausen and Kohn[36] has been extremely important in this area. Their studies suggest that downward drift, although important, does not fully account for the disproportionate number of lower class schizophrenic patients and that lower class living conditions do appear to play some role in the etiology of some schizophrenia. They have also provided a conceptual framework drawn from studies of social class, which could account for pathogenic effects of class on the vulnerable person. They hypothesize that, in contrast to the middle and upper classes, individuals in the lower classes generally are isolated from many community resources and have greater rigidity in their early environment, thus failing to develop a flexible repertoire for mastering problems. These conditions render persons from the lowest social class especially vulnerable to catastrophic decompensation in the face of stresses from high demands, weak support systems, or confusing social structures.

Although the social class findings have been replicated on many occasions, they have had little impact on research or clinical practice. Perhaps this is because the social class data are statistical results from large sample epidemiological studies difficult to apply to individual patients. It may also reflect the fact that influential research and clinical writing and teaching most often come from persons and institutions with predominantly upper and middle class orientations, while a large number of schizophrenic patients are lower class and unemployed.

Stressful Life Events

Psychosis is commonly observed to follow a life stress. But do such stresses have a role specifically in causing schizophrenia? If, in fact, stress is important in precipitating illness and its recurrence in schizophrenic patients, treatment and prevention implications are readily apparent.

We think stressful events do, at times, precipitate florid schizophrenic symptoms in vulnerable persons and that the clinician's effort to reduce stress, reduce vulnerability to stress, and dampen the impact of stress are wisely undertaken. However, this supposed cause-and-effect relationship is, in fact, very uncertain and difficult to document. Consider the following:

1. Assessment of life events and stress is an uncertain undertaking in normal populations, even with regard to stress-related illnesses such as hypertension. How, then, does one judge the stressful nature of events in a population of schizophrenic individuals so prone to idiosyncratic interpretations and reactions, responsivity to private phenomena, and dissociation of affect and cognition? The clinician may have to deal with this problem by making individualized judgments, while the investigator continues to grope for improved means of assessing life events with standardized methods.

2. It has almost become a truism that stress-precipitated psychotic episodes have a better prognosis than those unrelated to external events. This has not been easy to demonstrate with reliable methods but, if true, means that only a subpopulation of schizophrenic patients may have stress-precipitated disorders. This is conceptually important and may permit a meaningful subdivision of schizophrenia into stress-sensitive and "free-running" categories of illness. It must be remembered, however, that this latter category may be comprised of patients whose behavior is too deviant from social norms to be defined as stress-sensitive by standard methods, yet is quite stress-sensitive within their idiosyncratic framework. The patient who seems unperturbed by the death of a parent may become delusional in response to an airline crash in a distant city.

3. Early stages of decompensation are replete with stress and difficult life events. Whether these are judged to be precipitants of subsequent decompensation phases depends on the clinician's concept of the disease and skills as a phenomenologist. In our work together, we have often found it easy to agree on the presence or absence of stressful events but have found it difficult to agree on their role in pathogenesis.

Do stressful life events have an etiological role in schizophrenia? Many early studies, influenced perhaps by the belief that schizophrenia was an endogenous disorder unaffected by the environment, came to a negative answer. This suggested that, unlike many other types of psychopathology, the onset of schizophrenia was not much affected by life events. More recently, however, some investigations have suggested that, with finer measurement instruments and attention to the individual meaning of certain happenings, both onset and recurrence in schizo-phrenia may be considerably affected by stressful events.[37] The final answer is not in, but the pendulum appears to be swinging toward a suggestion that stressful life events may have an etiological role, do affect the course of disorder, and may also be of prognostic significance in schizophrenia.

A COMMENT ON PARADIGMS

The reader may have noted in comparing this chapter to the previous one how strikingly different the methodological issues are in studying biological and psychosocial etiologies. Although problems in assessment, measurement, diagnosis, sampling, and statistics are common to both efforts, for ethical and other reasons, psychosocial research tends to use naturalistic paradigms almost exclusively—observations of families with a schizophrenic member, reports of life events that have taken place, naturally occurring social class and cultural variations. The move from exclusively retrospective studies to more prospective models, as in risk research, has been an important one. Some experimental psychosocial research, as in certain studies by Reiss exploring how changes in the family members present impact on individual problem-solving, has also been introduced. But the full range of experimental research is not yet applicable to psychosocial studies. Development of more adequate re-search paradigms is clearly needed; at present, the limitations in research methods (and perhaps conception) discourage young investigators and research administrators from a concentrated focus on clarifying the role of psychosocial factors in schizophrenia.

SUMMARY

In considering the many psychological and social factors implicated in the etiology of schizophrenia, it is clear that important information is accumulating, information that discourages narrow theories and requires cross-disciplinary integration. Each domain may have a piece of the truth. Early childhood characteristics (especially those related to social be-havior), family characteristics (especially those involving communication patterns), characteristics of the larger social environment (especially labeling and social class), and stressful life events all appear to have etiological roles in schizophrenia. Each, however, appears to account for only some degree of likelihood that the disorder will occur, and then perhaps only in some patients. Because these findings suggest that a complex, multifactor etiology is involved, more knowledge about the power of each variable, its relationships to the others, and the development of improved models for understanding this process are important next steps in discovering the etiological pathways to schizophrenia.

RECOMMENDED READING

Burnham, D. L., Gladstone, A. I., and Gibson, R. W. *Schizophrenia and the need–fear dilemma.* New York: International Universities Press, 1969.

Chodoff, P., and Carpenter, W. T., Jr. Psychogenic theories of schizophrenia. In: *Schizophrenia: Biological and psychological perspectives,* Usdin, G. (ed.). New York: Brunner/Mazel, Inc., 1975.

Clausen, J., and Kohn, M. Relation of schizophrenia to the social structure of a small city. In: *Epidemiology of mental disorder.* Washington, D.C.: American Association for the Advancement of Science, 1969, 69–94.

Lidz, T. *The origin and treatment of schizophrenic disorders.* New York: Basic Books, Inc., 1973.

Strauss, J. S., Kokes, R. F., Klorman, R., and Sacksteder, J. Premorbid adjustment in schizophrenia: Concepts, measures and implications. *Schizophrenia Bulletin,* 1977, 3(2):182–244.

Watt, N. F. Patterns of childhood social development in adult schizophrenia. *Archives of General Psychiatry,* 1978, 35:160–165.

Wynne, L. C., and Singer, M. Thought disorder and family relations. *Archives of General Psychiatry,* 1963, 9:199–206.

REFERENCES

1. Chapman, L. J. Recent advances in the study of schizophrenic cognition. *Schizophrenia Bulletin,* 1979, 5:568–580.
2. Strauss, J. S., Kokes, R. F., Klorman, R., and Sacksteder, J. Premorbid adjustment in schizophrenia: Concepts, measures and implications. *Schizophrenia Bulletin,* 1977, 3(2):182–244.
3. Watt, N. F. Patterns of childhood social development in adult schizophrenia. *Archives of General Psychiatry,* 1978, 35:160–165.
4. Chodoff, P., and Carpenter, W. T., Jr. Psychogenic theories of schizophrenia. In: *Schizophrenia: Biological and psychological perspectives,* Usdin, G. (ed.). New York: Brunner/Mazel, Inc., 1975.

5. Klein, M. *Contributions to psychoanalysis, 1921-1945.* London: Hogarty Press, 1952.

6. Sullivan, H.S. *The interpersonal theory of psychiatry.* New York: Norton, 1953.

7. Hagen, R. Behavioral therapies and the treatment of schizophrenics. *Schizophrenia Bulletin,* 1975, 13:70–96.

8. Meyer, A. Fundamental conceptions of dementia praecox. In: *The commonsense psychiatry of Adolf Meyer,* Lief, A. New York: McGraw-Hill, 1948, 184–192.

9. Wise, C. D., Baden, M. M., and Stein L. Post mortem measurements of enzymes in human brain: Evidence of central noradrenergic deficit in schizophrenia. *Journal of Psychiatric Research,* 1974, 11:185–198.

10. Heston, L.L. The genetics of schizophrenia and schizoid disease. *Science,* 1970, 167:249–256.

11. Fromm-Reichmann, F. Notes on the development of treatment of schizophrenia by psychoanalytic psychotherapy. *Psychiatry,* 1948, 11:263–273.

12. Lidz, T., Fleck, S., and Cornelison, A. *Schizophrenia and the family.* New York: International Universities Press, 1965.

13. Bateson, G., Jackson, D., Haley, J., and Weakland, J. Towards a theory of schizophrenia. *Behavioral Science,* 1956, 1:251–264.

14. Berger, M. (ed.), *Beyond the double bind.* New York: Brunner/Mazel, 1978.

15. Wynne, L. C., and Singer, M. Thought disorder and family relations. *Archives of General Psychiatry,* 1963, 9:199–206.

16. Jones, J., Rodnick, E., Goldstein, M. *et al.* Parental transaction style deviance as a possible indicator of risk for schizophrenia. *Archives of General Psychiatry,* 1977, 34:71–74.

17. Hirsch, S., and Leff, J. *Abnormality in parents of schizophrenics.* London: Oxford University Press, 1975.

18. Woodward, J., and Goldstein, M. Communication deviance in the families of schizophrenics: A comment on the misuse of analysis of covariance. *Science,* 1977, 197:1096–1097.

19. Laing, R. *The politics of experience.* New York: Ballantine, 1967.

20. Wynne, L., Ryckoff, I., Day, J., and Hirsch, S. Pseudomutuality in the family relations of schizophrenics. *Psychiatry,* 1958, 21:205–220.

21. Reiss, D. Individual thinking and family interaction. *Journal of Nervous and Mental Disease,* 1969, 149:473–490.

22. Brown, G. W., Birley, J. L. T., and Wing, J. K. Influence of family life on the course of schizophrenic disorders: A replication. *British Journal of Psychiatry,* 1972, 121:241–258.

23. Vaughn, C. E., and Leff, J. P. The influence of family and social factors on the course of psychiatric illness: A comparison of schizophrenic and depressed neurotic patients. *British Journal of Psychiatry,* 1976, 129:125–137.

24. Leff, J. P. Schizophrenia and sensitivity to the family environment. *Schizophrenia Bulletin,* 1976, 2(4):566–574.

25. MacLean, P. The triune brain, emotion, and scientific bias. In: *The neurosciences second study program,* Schmitt, F.O. (ed.). New York: Rockefeller University Press, 1970.

26. Kreisman, D., and Joy, V. Family response to the mental illness of a relative. *Schizophrenia Bulletin*, 1974, 10:34–57.
27. Riskin, J., and Faunce, E. Family interaction scales. III. Discussion of methodology and substantive findings. *Archives of General Psychiatry*, 1970, 22:527–537.
28. Rosenhan, D. L. On being sane in insane places. *Science*, 1973, 179:250–257.
29. Caudill, W. *The psychiatric hospital as a small society*. Cambridge, MA: Harvard University Press, 1967.
30. Goffman, E. *Asylums*. Garden City, NY: Doubleday, 1961.
31. World Health Organization. *The international pilot study of schizophrenia*, vol. 1. Geneva: WHO Press, 1973.
32. Eaton, J., and Weil, R. *Culture and mental disorders*. Glencoe, IL: Free Press, 1955.
33. Murphy, H. Cultural influences on incidence, course, and treatment response. In: *The nature of schizophrenia*, Wynne, L., Cromwell, R., and Matthysse, S. (eds.). New York: Wiley, 1978.
34. Katz, M., Sanborn, K., Lowery, H., and Ching, J. Ethnic studies in Hawaii. In *The nature of schizophrenia*, Wynne, L., Cromwell, R., and Matthysse, S. (eds.). New York: Wiley, 1978.
35. World Health Organization. *Schizophrenia: An international follow-up study*. New York: Wiley, 1979.
36. Clausen, J. and Kohn, M. Relation of schizophrenia to the social structure of a small city. In: *Epidemiology of mental disorder*. Washington, D. C.: American Association for the Advancement of Science. 1969, 69–94.
37. Dohrenwend, B. S. & Dohrenwend, B. P. What is a stressful life event? In: *Guide to stress research*, Selye, H. (ed.). New York: VanNostrand, in press.

CHAPTER 9

Treatments

GENERAL PRINCIPLES

INTRODUCTION

Optimal treatment requires a clear identification of the disorder being treated and a comprehensive understanding of the sick person and his or her environment. But the enigmatic nature of schizophrenia makes this ideal difficult to realize. Understanding the illness, the setting in which it occurs, and the effects on the individual, requires time and skill. Even when such understanding is achieved, it does not assure decisive therapeutic intervention.

For these reasons, in many settings no reasonable attempt to achieve optimal treatment is even undertaken. In other settings, a narrow clinical or theoretical view of schizophrenia provides a pseudoclarity which encumbers the evaluation process with presuppositions, and treatment decisions follow theory rather than a careful description and understanding of the patient.

Many schools of thought compete to provide guidelines for understanding schizophrenia. Is schizophrenia a deficiency syndrome for which the treating clinician must substitute or replace that which is missing? Is schizophrenia a psychobiological reaction to be treated by removing the initiating factor or counterbalancing the altered biology? Is schizophrenia a human's complicated response to severe psychological conflict, such that anything less than conflict resolution is simply symptom suppression? Such basic questions remain essentially unanswered, although it is now apparent that none of these factors operates to the exclusion of the others.

Patient care, however, does not wait until definitive answers to questions about etiology, pathogenesis, diagnosis, and treatment have been given. Clinicians must act by observing, understanding, diagnosing, and treating the patient even in the absence of answers to these fundamental questions. The discussion of treatment to follow attempts to cope with these needs and gaps in knowledge by focusing on key treatment principles. Given the complexities involved, the discussion is simplified for sake of clarity. More details regarding specific treatment modalities and treatment questions will be provided in the following chapter. Although we will describe our understanding of the many things now known about treating schizophrenic patients, the definitive answers, however desirable and sought for, cannot be supplied at this time.

THE CLINICAL CONTEXT FOR TREATING THE PERSON

The core of treatment is the interpersonal context. In order to obtain information for diagnosis and treatment planning, the clinician must be extensively involved as participant–observer. Ancillary aids to diagnosis are desirable, but the clinician cannot intelligently formulate meaning and type of psychopathology or put forward a comprehensive therapeutic approach without an intimate professional involvement. Similarly, the patient is not to be viewed as a passive receptacle of treatment but is to be involved (psychopathology notwithstanding!) in providing information, conceptualizing treatment, becoming informed, and granting or denying consent to interventions. Besides its importance for diagnosis and treatment planning, the clinical relationship, from the very beginning, also provides the initial therapeutic impact.

To meet these needs, starting with the first clinical encounter, five major issues are important: security, contact, psychological insight, collaboration, and establishing expectations. The reader may recall the patient described in previous chapters as these points are elaborated.

Security

During periods of psychosis, patients are often frightened and/or frightening; establishing security for the patient and clinician, therefore, is of prime importance. Even when bodily safety is not at issue, unpredictable and strange behavior may be intimidating. A physical setting providing reasonable comfort to patient *and* clinician is required. Arranging for an interview room free of dangerous objects, the presence of other staff or a family member, and an open door are examples of steps that can be taken to reduce patient and clinician anxiety. Efforts aimed at providing control usually require an explanatory comment to the patient (e.g., "I want others present while we talk so that I can be less concerned about myself and more attentive to what you say"). Candor and clarification may reduce the patient's apprehension and sense of isolation and help the patient understand the context of the situation. If security is not achieved, the clinician may hide behind a mask of professionalism or neutrality and unwittingly avoid issues that are important but might increase anxiety.

When problems of control require more dramatic intervention, the interpersonal context permits individualized rather than stereotyped responses. Large doses of injected medication or physical restraints are too often utilized as alternatives to the simple, direct approach described above. The extreme methods are legitimate for management in acute cases, but decisions about their use should, whenever possible, emerge from the interpersonal context, not replace it. In establishing safety, techniques which decrease violence with maximum collaboration of patient and clinician have priority.

Contact

Schizophrenic patients often experience a pervasive sense of isolation. Several illness-related factors are involved: (a) the patient's subjective experiences may be so bizarre, primitive, or troublesome that he feels he is different from others—particularly those who seem relaxed and able to oganize their thinking and to pursue goals without a flood of impulses and thoughts; (b) the patient's behavior may cause others to distance themselves or to respond in a way emphasizing to the patient that he is different; (c) many schizophrenic patients have a basic impairment in their ability to establish rapport and maintain a social network; and (d) the patient is often removed from his natural setting and placed in a clinical environment devoid of the ordinary reminders of his interpersonal ties.

The clinician working with the schizophrenic patient needs to be particularly aware of the importance of facilitating nonintrusive interpersonal contact and of avoiding dehumanizing processes wherever possible. This is a difficult task, for the violent, agitated, or bizarre patient drives others away; the socially withdrawn patient fails to provide the ordinary gratifications of personal contact; the distracted, dissociated patient frustrates efforts at communication; and stereotyped role expectations that may be assumed by clinician and patient tend to insulate the patient from ordinary human interactions.

For these reasons, it is especially important that the clinician establish and maintain a professionally expressed personal involvement with the patient. The clinician should not be overly intrusive and impatient and should not deemphasize the clinician's role by substituting a pseudofriendliness and informality. It is important, however, that clinicians not depersonalize their relationship with patients by resorting to stereotyped behavior emulating the aloof, authoritarian doctor and minimizing empathic communication.

History-taking, for example, can be a process mutually informative to patient and clinician, enhancing the therapeutic relationship. On the other hand, there is a style of history-taking which seeks specific facts with little interest in the individual's experience. This dehumanizing approach may serve to reduce the clinician's anxiety with a psychotic patient, but it will convince the patient that he will be frustrated in any effort to have his highly charged personal experiences taken seriously by his clinician.

When initially evaluating a schizophrenic patient, the clinician may unthinkingly neglect ordinary inquiries. If a patient is dissociated in his thinking and disordered in behavior, we may not ask him why he has come to the hospital. The answer seems obvious, and other informants are more precise. But to bypass the patient already suggests that we devalue his view of events, are impatient with his capacity to communicate, and do not find direct assessment of his subjective experiences important for our clinical task.

Another consideration at the outset is clarification of our role. The clinician needs to appreciate the patient's expectations and wishes in this regard. Many patients will have been told by others what to expect from us. Since the clinician's view of his role may not fit with the patient's or family's expectations, it is important that these views be discussed. The clinician can state clearly and simply that his role is to determine whether aspects of the patient's functioning suggest that he has a psychiatric problem and if so, to formulate diagnosis and treatment.

The initial interviews focus on data pertaining to the presenting problem, history, social context, and the diagnostic axes. Process as well as content should be noticed and, when necessary, discussed, since the "feel" of the interview often provides important clues to the patient's problems. Some of these may already be causing obstacles to the evaluation itself. For example, the patient without insight may feel coerced and respond, "I don't know," to many queries. "Did someone else make you come to the hospital?" followed by "What bothered them?" may alter the process sufficiently to permit the patient to become informative and feel that the interviewer is helpful. Often, clinicians inexperienced in working with schizophrenic patients are hesitant to shift the process away from the "I'm a doctor, you're a patient" format, but an early stalemate may be sidestepped by exploring from the patient's point of view. This does not subvert clinician and patient roles but emphasizes the patient's vantage as legitimate.

In the initial interviews, it is important to find a balance between the patient's self-declared boundaries and the clinician's need for information. For example, if inquiries about delusions provoke defensiveness, one can note out loud that it is troublesome to talk about these things and that it may be best to move to another topic for the time being. It is often more productive to allow time to follow the patient's lead rather than attempt to impose a predetermined format on the initial interview. In structured research interviews, we find that a few minutes of nondirective interviewing at the start establishes a tone or process that permits many specific questions to be pursued. Schizophrenic patients, like everyone else, can talk better when they are being listened to.

The tendency to ignore or rationalize even the most profound processes occurring between patient and clinician is manifest in many ways. Some clinicians believe schizophrenics too fragile to be "confronted" with the consequences of their behavior or to discuss their internal experience. Some clinicians may feel bored to the point of being inattentive or may proceed with orderly inquiries but avoid mentioning a patient's confusing or intimidating behavior. At times, the operating assumption seems to be that to note a type of behavior is to cause or magnify it. Imagine how isolating it would be to have our own behavior go unnoted by those around us.

Often simply mentioning important aspects of the interaction between patient and clinician can provide a basis of shared experience which serves as a building block for a therapeutic alliance. And such processes or the consequences of a patient's behavior can be discussed without being provocative or becoming preoccupied with the issues being noted. The attitude of "let sleeping dogs lie" is often misused with schizophrenic patients. To be sure, dormant conflict-ridden material is sometimes inappropriately evoked by the interviewer; but more often the patient cannot escape primitive thoughts and impulses, yet the clinician suggests directly or indicates in some fashion that such material should not be dealt with in the evaluation session.

Comments on the process of the interview are sometimes difficult to make even if the problems involved are obvious. For example, a Spanish-speaking patient was difficult to understand and appeared to comprehend little of what was discussed in spite of the fact that she was fluent in English. Nothing was said on this topic until a consultant interviewed this patient and, after about two minutes with her, asked, "You speak with a very heavy Spanish accent; why is that?" This simple comment provoked a discussion which indicated that this woman was using the Spanish accent and her apparent difficulty in understanding English to avoid interaction with those around her. In our experience, when such obvious factors are ignored, the isolation of the schizophrenic patient is increased and the clinician's ability to become familiar with his patient's inner world is impaired.

Psychological Insight

The personal experience of schizophrenic illness is a crisis which contains the seeds for growth as well as the potential for deterioration. This is true regardless of the etiology and pathogenesis of the illness, since the content of psychotic experience is personal and may be richly informative. As with dreams, the form of expression in psychosis may be the same from individual to individual, but the content is idiosyncratic and informative concerning the individual's past experiences and psychological conflicts. Some material is highly symbolic, and careful attention to the development and expression of symptomatology, the social setting in which it occurs, and the patient's associations with this material can provide a basis for meaningful insights into the patient's psychology.

We believe it is a mistake to view schizophrenia as a desirable stage of conflict resolution, and to espouse the schizophrenic experience as an existential accomplishment is to ignore the terrible toll on human potential caused by this disorder. However, patients need to achieve a perspective about the content of their illness; it is wasteful when we fail to provide the psychotic patient with an opportunity to learn about himself during a perplexing yet informative personal crisis.

The extent to which this potential can be utilized depends on the interest and capabilities of the patient and clinician. Some patients, whether schizophrenic or not, have strong personal tendencies toward denial and encapsulation which may make them poor subjects for psychological exploration and integration of experiences. With such patients, an effort to provide some personal framework for understanding aspects of their symptomatology may go only far enough to supply a basis for a collaborative therapeutic relationship with sufficient insight into illness to cooperate in future treatment endeavors, recognize early signs of impending episodes, and identify factors producing decompensation which might be resolved or avoided.

In contrast, many people, including schizophrenic patients, have a personal propensity toward introspection and self-understanding. For patients who have this propensity, it provides a basis for psychological therapy both during and following psychotic episodes. With these patients, psychotherapeutic goals will go beyond an acknowledgement of illness and the identification of aspects of illness critical to a treatment collaboration. The patient will tend to explore his experiences, and the techniques and perspective of his therapist can further this exploration.

It is a natural human tendency to provide an explanatory framework for personal crises, but it is important in schizophrenia to avoid premature or distorted closure. The process of examining the details of decompensation and recompensation provides the patient with a basis for identifying vulnerabilities, reducing distortions, and developing a sense of personal mastery in the face of psychotic experiences. An exploration of these experiences with the clinician provides the optimal setting for developing a therapeutic relationship and obtaining information critical to decision-making on a broad range of treatment issues.

It is not known whether an integrating or sealing-over recovery is best in terms of subsequent course.[1,2] We believe that most patients will follow their personal proclivities in this regard. However, for patients inclined toward integrating their experiences, the goal of fostering such insight should be considered.

Collaboration

Collaboration between clinician and patient should begin at the first contact; such collaboration is difficult to achieve later if it is ignored early. This point should not require discussion, but so many patients describe their treatment experiences as devoid of collaboration, and service delivery mechanisms pose so many impediments to early collaboration, that comment is required. Many patients who become psychotic find, for example, that an initial and major treatment decision (initiation of pharmacotherapy) is made prior to any effort at understanding their experiences and is clearly based on concepts of the illness rather than on an individualized clinical decision. From a clinician's point of view, we would further complain that major treatment decisions are often made in advance of careful diagnosis, with no broad appreciation of the patient's strengths and weaknesses, and no opportunity for the patient to understand the basis of the treatment formulation.

The collaborative orientation to treatment implies that patient and clinician work together to achieve therapeutic success. Such an orientation can be pursued even with a violent, paranoid, or involuntary patient. Collaboration is a general approach implying neither the abdication of the clinician's authority and expertise nor the postponement of therapeutic decisions until there is mutuality concerning them. Collaboration only requires that the clinician continuously involve the patient in the information base from which treatment decisions emerge, that the patient be given ample opportunity to understand, contribute to, and consent to treatment, and that the patient be told the basis for any decision to proceed with treatment against his wishes. This ideal can be pursued by the clinician even when the patient is unable or unwilling to collaborate.

The assumption that the patient cannot participate in a collaborative relationship leads many clinicians to initiate treatment without attempting to understand the patient's experience or to communicate the treatment rationale. Patients may first hear about medication from nursing staff who have the responsibility of giving it, and the explanation may be only that "Your doctor thinks you should have this." Such a comment is quite different from a doctor's explaining to a patient the reasons for giving medications and even, when necessary, why medication is being provided before it is mutually agreed upon or the patient's condition thoroughly understood.

We make no pretense that patients always understand or communicate rationally about these matters, but it is the physician's responsibility to provide the patient with every opportunity to participate, even when the patient is only minimally able to do so. Furthermore, we are often surprised when a few weeks or months later patients recall in detail the initial discussions. A patient who insists that we are trying to poison him or destroy his sexual organs may simultaneously be struggling to grasp the helping nature of our intervention.

The collaborative approach is also crucial in deciding what to treat. In the beginning, clinical emergencies and urgencies may require that we start treatment before being fully informed about the breadth of the patient's dysfunction or the sustaining strengths on which we may capitalize. Many patients, however, are far more communicative in the initial phases and provide the clinician an opportunity to consider a broad range of psychopathology and possible degrees of competence as treatment recommendations are conceptualized. The collaborative relationship provides an opportunity for the clinician to present to the patient his formulation and treatment recommendations and to describe for the patient the major concerns, expectations of treatment, and, in the mutually informative interchange, to define new areas for treatment consideration.

Expectations

Wittingly or not, the patient, family, employers, clinicians, and other elements of society are continually setting expectations which influence the course of illness. If psychosis is interpreted as a permanent disability, the patient's future work accomplishments will be curtailed. If psychotic behavior is interpreted as voluntary belligerence aimed at avoiding responsibility, the patient may be pressured to assume functions beyond his ability to cope. The clinician needs to make early clarification of an optimal level of expectations, even though rapid change in the optimal level might be expected. Taking care of a patient to such a degree that a passive role is fostered minimizes the patient's opportunity to demonstrate and observe his own strengths. Caring for an ill individual and at the same time trying to reduce one's personal anxiety often cause clinical staffs and families to lower expectations of the patient unwisely. Some patients require "total care," at least during some phases of illness, and symptomatic exacerbations can result from unrealistically high expectations. However, low expectations, especially during early stages of illness, may reinforce the patient's reduced self-esteem and complicate recovery, with premature closure on helplessness.

In the clinician/patient dyad, clarification of the clinician's expectations is necessary, and he should also encourage the patient to participate actively in deciding what expectations are reasonable. One must consider that the patient may be informative, that the patient may participate in identifying some common basis for the clinical relationship, that the patient may exert some degree of control over his behavior, and that the patient may identify areas of special vulnerability to assist the clinical staff in providing appropriate care.

Later in treatment, following at least partial symptomatic recovery from a psychotic episode, defining expectations will require attention to the more enduring and socially relevant aspects of the patient's functioning capability. The patient faces questions of whether he can work and, if so, at what level; whether to attempt to maintain family relationships and to establish social contacts outside of the home, and many other problems involved in the ordinary pursuit of life. Unrealistically high expectations may be stressful and make the patient more vulnerable to decompensation; unnecessarily low expectations, on the other hand, may lead to an increasingly constricted life.

The clinician's best judgment about reasonable expectations must be articulated clearly to the patient, but most important is a shared understanding of the basis for reaching such judgments. Clinicians cannot attain such a basis without intimate familiarity with the patient's strengths and limitations in the broadest range of intrapsychic and interpersonal functioning. Those who treat schizophrenic patients sometimes have a tendency to make sweeping generalizations concerning expectations (e.g., schizophrenic patients relapse if pushed to get jobs) without benefit of an individualized assessment of the patient's strengths. Furthermore, because a patient's capabilities will shift radically from one phase of illness to another, defining expectations must be a fluid process. This view is reinforced by the fact that schizophrenia is a heterogeneous syndrome and that functional capability is not determined solely by the illness. The clinician must consider not only the disorder itself, but each patient's innate strengths and the social environment as well.

When patients can be treated with continuity by the individuals providing care, one can be less concerned with the risk of setting expectations too high. Not only will the clinician become better informed as contacts with the patient involve all phases of illness and recovery, but the risk of psychotic decompensation can be minimized when early detection and rapid treatment are possible. With present techniques, we are far more effective in the treatment of psychotic exacerbations than in the alteration of deficit functioning. Hence, the capacity to utilize brief hospital stays or targeted drug treatment can be reassuring when the clinician and the patient take some risk in setting expectations which may be difficult for the patient to achieve.

PROCESSES REQUIRING TREATMENT ATTENTION

From the contextual issues of treatment described above, it is now possible to proceed to general guidelines for treating specific areas of dysfunction. Each person will present many individual characteristics of therapeutic relevance, but there are a few major areas of human functioning which routinely require attention in the evaluation and treatment of schizophrenic patients. These areas can be represented diagnostically and conceptually as "axes." In considering treatment, special attention is placed on five such axes and the processes they represent: symptomatology, course, associated or precipitating factors, social and family relationship functioning, and work or "primary role" functioning.

Symptomatology

The treatment of symptoms in the schizophrenic patient receives particular emphasis, since symptom manifestations are generally what bring the patient to the clinician's attention. Medication and psychotherapy have been viewed as alternative approaches for ameliorating symptoms, but a broader range of treatment modalities has the potential to reduce symptoms, and some combination of therapies is usually indicated.

Two difficulties complicate the choice of treatment for symptom reduction. The first of these is the existence of several types of symptoms. It is convenient to divide symptoms into positive and negative types, using the precedent set by Hughlings Jackson.[3] Delusions and hallucinations are examples of positive symptoms. Apathy and restricted affect are examples of negative symptoms. A third type of symptom, "dysphoric" symptoms, such as depression and anxiety, can also be identified.[4] Given several discrete symptom dimensions, should treatment strategy attend specifically to each type?

The second complication in considering symptom treatment arises from the question of what is central to the schizophrenic disorder. In the past especially, some clinicians focused on psychodynamic processes and viewed drug-induced symptom reduction as chemical interference with resolution of underlying conflict. Other clinicians have focused on somatic concepts of schizophrenia and have relied exclusively on pharmacotherapy for treatment. A happier day is at hand now that the severe limitations of each treatment modality are being thrown into clear relief and multifactorial therapeutic concepts encourage treatment innovations.

The issues of symptom type and treatment focus complicate therapeutic decisions because they arise from basic unanswered questions about the "true" nature of schizophrenia. While awaiting the resolution of those basic questions, the clinician may combine and balance various treatment strategies aimed at symptom reduction.

Approaches to these strategies will be illustrated in the next chapter, but one general point must be made here. Use of antipsychotic medications for symptom reduction and prevention merits special attention because their therapeutic efficacy is clearly established, their use is ubiquitous, and their administration can be precisely defined. Two common problems in the pharmacotherapy of schizophrenia also deserve mention—selection of patients and timing of intervention. It is natural for the clinician to wish to relieve pain as soon as possible. However, as in other fields of medicine, immediate symptom relief may not be the optimal treatment. There are good reasons why morphine is withheld until a patient with acute abdominal pain is diagnosed. Ordinary practice today with psychotic patients seems based on the assumption that only one course of action is available and ignores the importance of diagnosis and the need to derive treatment decisions from a broad base of information.

If drug therapy is to be carried out most effectively, timing of intervention is important. Drugs may be beneficial in some phases of illness without being required in all. In the initiation of pharmacotherapy, the social and psychological connotations of intervention must also be considered. A terrified paranoid patient suffers from anxiety, but some elements of the psychotic experience may be gratifying or reassuring. We have seen, for example, patients who have woven such an elaborate paranoid frame of reference that they were enthralled with the intrigue of constant danger and surprise. To alleviate their apprehension immediately was to misunderstand the important self-perpetuating gratifications involved. With other patients, hallucinatory experiences were reported as uncomfortable, but removing the hallucinations was associated with a sense of loss and abandonment.

Some patients actually induce psychotic symptoms. One patient experienced continuous and dysphoric visual and auditory hallucinations. When high-dose antipsychotic medication was given, the intensity and frequency of the hallucinatory experiences were rapidly reduced, but the patient was then observed standing in the solarium staring at the sun. When asked why, he explained that staring at the sun reactivated the hallucinations. This patient had to be physically restrained to prevent his staring at the sun; at the same time, we talked with him further to determine why the hallucinations were so important.

The point is a simple one: Treatment of symptoms—as treatment of any aspect of disorder—is best carried out from the broadest possible information base. A too rapid and too "heroic" use of antipsychotic medication in treating the symptoms of schizophrenia may interfere with obtaining such a broad base, and treatment interventions may prevent adequate patient collaboration.

Course of Disorder

The second axis or process with treatment implications is the course of illness. The idea of treating the course of a disorder (in contrast to altering its future evolution) may appear strange, since we usually think of the course of an illness as its unfolding pattern and try mainly to prevent untoward developments. A subtle but important distinction is to regard course as the longitudinal manifestation of illness requiring active therapy in its own right.

Each type of course found in schizophrenia requires particular treatment considerations. For example, the possibility of chronicity and deterioration requires special attention to problems of hospitalization and pharmacological treatment. The chronic use of hospitals and drugs, singly or in combination, has many dangers. Institutions for long-term treatment are often more custodial than therapeutic, and the psychosocial impact of chronic institutionalization may interact negatively with the illness to produce profound mental deterioration. Major therapeutic impetus currently involves the movement to deinstitutionalize patients and provide community support and maintenance antipsychotic medication.

But the chronic use of antipsychotic drugs also presents problems, since it is associated with a high risk of neurological complications, may induce apathy or anhedonia, or interact negatively in other ways with the effects of chronic illness. The prophylactic use of maintenance anti-psychotic medication has been an extremely important development, and it is clearly established that patients vulnerable to an episodic course of illness will receive partial protection from relapse through such treatment. However, the frequent assumption of chronicity in schizophrenia has generated the consequent failure to be careful in limiting the use of antipsychotic medication to patients who have demonstrated a chronic or episodic course. Many acute nonepisodic patients are continued on medication despite risk and without clear indication of therapeutic efficacy. Similarly, many chronic patients are no longer episodic, and prophylactic medication in these patients is no longer justified. In fact, careful attention to course suggests that there are several treatment-relevant subtypes of schizophrenia.[5]

In many instances, we are hard pressed to find better alternatives for extensive hospitalization and/or long-term pharmacotherapy, since community-based care has proved to be a myth for many patients.[6] It is becoming increasingly clear, however, that treating chronic course of disorder adequately requires therapeutic hospitals and judicious pharmacotherapy, as well as the development of better access to psychosocial treatments, community living, and occupational programs.

The course of disorder also has a major interaction with the patient's environment which must be dealt with. It has been shown, for example,[7] that after a patient has been rehospitalized on three occasions or more, the family tends to become discouraged and to detach itself. The patient is set adrift. Work with the patient and the family around this problem may help to mitigate some of the negative consequences of such a chain of events.

There is yet another sense in which the course of disorder requires attention in treatment planning. Treatment varies depending on the phase of disorder. The treatment required during a period of florid psychosis, postpsychotic depression, partial remission, or after several recurrences may involve different applications of interpersonal, pharmacological, and rehabilitation modalities. Awareness of this obvious but often neglected fact must alert the clinician to the need for flexibility in the treatment program. The variable and often complex course of schizophrenia only serves further to emphasize that there is not *a* treatment for schizophrenia, but rather an armamentarium of treatment modalities that must be tailored to the individual's situation.

It is especially important in considering the phase of disorder to draw a sharp distinction between management required in an emergency situation and treatment required for prolonged periods. This distinction is necessary to prevent the assumption that an intervention which has profound effect in an emergency is, therefore, a necessary component of future treatment. Just because a flagrantly disturbed patient may become calm when physically separated from the social setting in which he became psychotic, the clinician would hardly conclude automatically that indefinite separation from that social setting is an essential component of further treatment. Similarly, although the clinician may consider a quiet room or other diminution of social stimuli important in certain specified circumstances, he would hardly conclude that it is necessary for the patient to continue in that situation as an essential component of long-term treatment. The emergency use of antipsychotic medication can also achieve a valuable calming effect when needed, but this management strategy should not be presumed to indicate a need for further such treatment. Clinicians generally do not confuse the first two circumstances, but it has become commonplace to assume that an emergency room patient who receives antipsychotic medication and calms down must have a drug-responsive illness requiring continued treatment with the drug.

Associated Events

Associated or precipitating events are important considerations in treatment for two reasons. To the extent that such life events are precipitants of the patient's symptoms or social dysfunction, they reflect stresses that he or she will need to recognize. The possible impact on the patient of losses, physical illness, and difficult family or job situations are all factors that must be considered by the clinician so that psychotherapeutic treatment, medication change, environmental alterations, or other steps can be focused on helping the patient learn to cope with or avoid such situations or to overcome vulnerability to these stresses.

Understanding associated events may also help in evaluating etiological factors in the patient's disorder. It is possible, for example, to explore the background of certain particularly stressful events in order to help both patient and clinician understand these processes better and develop better modes of dealing with them. Especially with bizarre symptoms, such as delusions or hallucinations, establishing ties with life events can help to render the schizophrenic experience less mysterious and frightening and also to make the patient feel more human and less isolated.

Social Relationships

Problems with social relationships, especially with self–other boundaries, closeness, and isolation, are often considered hallmarks of schizophrenia. Even clinicians not viewing social relations dysfunction as diagnostically important generally accept the fact that a basic problem in the course of schizophrenia is social isolation and withdrawal. To deal with these problems, several treatment approaches are available. How they are used depends considerably on the type and seriousness of the social relations dysfunction as well as on the availability of skilled clinicians. Since schizophrenic patients may come from disturbed or disadvantaged family settings, it is important to evaluate these settings and consider ways in which a difficult environment might be modified to benefit the patient. If modification appears impossible, the clinician can use a clear understanding of the situation in which the schizophrenic patient lives in such a way that insight, sympathy, exhortation, or other approaches can be used with the patient on a realistic basis.

Psychotherapy—individual, group, or family—may help the patient learn about his patterns in relating and sources of mistrust and alienation. With these modalities, which will be discussed in more detail in Chapter 10, it is possible to help clarify which fears and patterns of relating are appropriate and which are maladaptive.

Another major treatment approach for helping the patient improve the ability to relate is social skills training. Several methods for this have been developed. Which one is used depends partly on the degree of the patient's disability[8,9] and on the programs available. Research reports have demonstrated the value of these approaches, and many patients spontaneously describe their usefulness. Because, unfortunately, social skills training is sometimes seen as "merely" rehabilitation or as outside the narrow version of the medical model, it has been difficult to obtain support for such treatment in many clinical settings.

Occupational Function

About two-thirds of schizophrenic patients are unemployed. Although for some patients work is an area of function that remains intact in spite of symptoms and social relations problems, many patients have difficulty with motivation, with their employers, with work habits, or with the stresses of occupational success or failure. Patients requiring frequent hospitalization may find it especially difficult to return to work and withstand the associated embarrassment and shame. Impairment in initiative, motivation, motor dexterity, and social skills may place schizophrenic patients at a particular employment disadvantage.

To help with these difficulties, vocational rehabilitation programs are included in many clinical settings. However, their integration into the needs of mental health programs continues to pose many serious problems.[10] Much remains to be learned about the optimal linking of vocational and other treatment programs, about establishing expectations of patient function that are neither too low nor too high, and about evaluating and responding to the changing amounts of stress with which patients are able to cope. Some of the most successful programs are independent of medically oriented care (e.g., Fountain House), perhaps because of continuing conceptual, practical, and territorial–professional problems in fully integrating treatment of disease and promotion of competence.

IMPLICATIONS OF FOCUSING TREATMENT ON THE FIVE PROCESSES

By focusing on several disordered processes, it is possible to avoid the reductionism and subsequent polarization that has so often marked approaches to the treatment of schizophrenia. Believing that drug and psychosocial treatments are mutually exclusive, for example, makes no sense in this context. Rather than viewing any treatment modality as focusing on the whole disease, considering various functional processes that require specific treatment planning fosters flexibility and empiricism in selecting treatment strategies.

Implementation of the multiple process approach to treatment requires reevaluation of some current beliefs.[11] It challenges, for example, the "common knowledge" that floridly psychotic patients must receive antipsychotic drugs as soon as they enter clinical care (e.g., in the emergency room) and emphasizes instead the need for thorough diagnostic evaluation and the establishment of a clinical relationship before treatment is begun whenever possible—and it usually is possible. The frequent pressures for instant treatment, although understandable, create an almost exclusive focus on positive symptoms. When these pressures combine with further undue pressures for rapid discharge from the hospital, the setting for a careful phenomenological assessment and personalized therapeutic intervention may never materialize.

The decline in use of interpersonal clinical strategies in the care of psychotic patients is partly based on problems in demonstrating their therapeutic efficacy. Although this may be relevant to psychotherapeutic attempts at symptom reduction, it does not relate to the interpersonal basis of clinical care generally, for evaluation, or for specific goals in other therapeutically relevant axes.

We argue that the clinician's personal involvement is crucial even on purely phenomenological grounds—there is no other method available for understanding and fully describing a patient's experience—and on clinical/humanitarian grounds—the strength of a therapeutic alliance in the treatment and healing process. It is peculiar that these principles are questioned vigorously in psychiatry, while the doctor/patient relationship is accepted as a critical ingredient in the therapeutic efficacy of somatic and pharmacological treatments in so many other specialties.

OTHER CONSIDERATIONS

Support for the Clinician

There is an unfortunate bravado sometimes associated with assuming responsibility for therapeutic interventions. At the extreme, this involves the reckless abandon exercised by undisciplined professionals who vigorously pursue the task of changing individuals without taking on the ordinary longitudinal role of a responsible clinician. Very often, such attempts are supported by uncritical assessments of success, and a failure to note untoward consequences.

Work with psychotic patients is undermined by such bravado, for the mechanisms of denial and insensitivity, which may at times be useful in more technological approaches to care, preclude the interpersonal aspects of treatment so important for work with a psychotic person.

To be interested in, care for, and understand a psychotic patient, it is necessary for the clinician to come face to face with the most perplexing and provocative human emotion and thought. It is natural for anyone, including the physician, to shield oneself from the impulsivity and primary process involved in relating with a psychotic person. But an important thread running through this book is a caution to the clinician about the potential antidiagnostic and antitherapeutic aspects of this shielding.

To succeed in the participant–observer role necessary for understanding the inner world of the psychotic person, a clinical environment truly supportive of clinical observation and of informed, individualized treatment is required. This does not negate the importance of security, control, and rapid decision-making, but it places behavioral control and symptom eradication in a broad clinical context rather than encouraging an exclusive focus on the symptom axes.

Such supportive settings are rare. When a heart patient develops edema, we first assume cardiac dysfunction and only secondarily question whether shortcomings in treatment account for the dysfunction. The reverse often occurs in psychiatry, and once a patient enters treatment, whatever goes wrong is presumed to reflect the shortcomings of the clinician and only secondarily is considered a consequence of illness. The clinician responsible for the treatment of psychotic patients is often personally held responsible for limits in the effectiveness of treatment. The cumulative impact is to force clinical care into carefully circumscribed behavior which seems beyond the reproach of peers and ignores the fundamental fact that we are dealing with a severe illness for which there is no definitive treatment.

The undermining of the clinician's role is often formalized. In some settings, the clinician is held responsible for any aggressive act which takes place in an unmedicated patient, as though aggressive acts never took place in medicated patients; similarly, in peer review he may be required to explain his failure to discharge the schizophrenic patient within 21 days.

A hopeful sign for psychiatry's future is the renewed interest in the severely ill and the challenge of the complex concepts necessary to synthesize information relevant to schizophrenia. This direction will be favored by open minded support provided for treatment and research endeavors that do not fit within a narrow, stereotyped model. If clinical institutions can provide supportive administrative, legal, social, and professional attitudes, increasing numbers of the most thoroughly qualified psychiatrists will assume responsibility for the care and study of psychotic patients, and more gifted clinical scientists will devote their energies to unravelling the puzzle of schizophrenia.

While progress in attracting clinicians and investigators to the problems of schizophrenia may depend on increasingly sympathetic attitudes, intellectual appreciation of the issues involved, and sociopolitical factors in psychiatry, it is also important to mention that the personal rewards and gratification of providing clinical care for the schizophrenic patient can be enormous. Patients change over time for better and worse; the clinician can make a difference and is constantly faced with new challenges in the necessity for acting with incomplete knowledge. We cannot avoid the sadness and despair associated with the mental and social deterioration of many schizophrenic patients, nor the anger and frustration associated with maintaining a therapeutic stance in the face of negativity, apathy, hate, the wish to die, or inability to experience the ordinary gratifications of relating to another person. But there is also the deep satisfaction of seeing a severely disordered person establish a rewarding life and the pleasure of assisting in that process.

Pressure to Act: Precipitous Action and Premature Closure

It is important for the clinician to remain cognizant of the fact that, in the face of psychotic phenomena, the patient, family, clinicians, and society are uncomfortable, press for action, and are vulnerable to premature closure on many issues. The pressure is understandable, but it is only partially accounted for by clinical necessity. We have already discussed some individual attributes of the psychotic patient that require exploration rather than precipitous action. But beyond these, clinical staffs often tend to subscribe to rather uniform principles of immediate care and management, and the individual clinician must conform or experience dissonance and the threat of exclusion from the group. These unwitting forces are powerful and conflict with the clinician's belief that he is free to make whatever decisions he judges to be in the best interest of the patient.

The common uniformity of treatment despite patient heterogeneity may reflect the extent to which covert assumptions and group expectations influence clinical care. Physicians in training are particularly aware of these problems. They note, for example, that their training will be completed without their ever having seen a diagnosed schizophrenic patient off medication. If they attempt to spend the first few hours or several days of hospital care evaluating a patient prior to administering drugs, there may be insistence from the staff that they provide "ethical and necessary" treatment. Senior supervisors and primary physicians may be so accustomed to these constraints that they teach a rigidly prescribed management regimen for the acutely psychotic patient.

Families also press for action. Their insistent belief that the patient must be medicated, must be hospitalized, must remain in a chronic care institution, or must return to their home rather than live independently is often difficult for patient and clinician to evaluate. The family has a compelling perspective on the effects of the illness, shares the burden, and may make legitimate claims to have its own needs met in clinical care decisions. The clinician may find it difficult to acknowledge the claims and receive information from families while simultaneously using his expertise on family attributes relevant to illness and treatment. However, attention to factors such as the putative pathogenic role of parental communication deviance,[12] the impact of expressed emotion in families on relapse and pharmacotherapeutic needs,[13] and the tendency of families to reach premature closure on key issues[14] require the clinician to resist pressures to act hastily.

In one instance, for example, a 20-year-old chronic schizophrenic man was admitted to a general hospital psychiatric ward for the purpose of being transferred for "indefinite stay" to a state hospital. The ward physician felt he was simply assigned the task of committing the patient and that evaluation, reconceptualization of the problem, and otherwise thinking creatively as a clinician were not expected. As he reflected on this later, the clinician felt that some of the impetus for the indefinite stay prescription came from within, but he could also identify points of pressure from the staff and from the patient's family. The patient did little to encourage a fresh consideration of his problems, since he remained mute and passive, manifested bizarre behavior, and was inappropriate in the social context of the unit. In this instance, the clinician sought a two-week period to evaluate the patient and arrive at therapeutic plans. By the end of this period, he had decided against transferring the patient to a state hospital; by the time of discharge, the patient had achieved a higher level of functioning and better quality of living than at any time in his recent past, higher than had been thought possible by many staff members or the family.

We have gone to some length on this point because it is so difficult for the individual clinician to recognize and resist pressures to conform to predefined expectations. Clues to such a situation are the clinician's feelings of pressure to act or of having no choice. Exploration of the situation often shows many incongruous phenomena. Although it might appear that something needs to be accomplished definitively in a day or two, neither the therapeutic nor financial considerations may actually require such a time limit. Once such a situation is recognized, the sources of felt pressure can be identified and the clinician can take a counteroffensive to determine from the patient, family, and others why they feel so much pressure. This turnabout is helpful not only in providing more rational treatment planning but in exposing important psychological issues central to the patient's problem and to his milieu.

Similar pressures occur in other settings as well, for example, in emergency rooms where psychotic patients are routinely medicated prior to transfer to an inpatient unit. In these and other instances, a major clue is the use of homogeneous treatment prescription, warning signs that essential steps of thorough assessment and the consideration of multifocal treatment strategies are not taking place.

Service Delivery

In the administration of health services, concepts of triage and allocation of resources have been influential in establishing the circumstances for treating schizophrenic patients. Triage may be useful and economical when resources are short, and selecting cases for intensive intervention may be particularly important. Employing such principles, health care administrators have played a useful role in providing services to a broader range of patients, especially the poverty-stricken schizophrenic person living in the community.

Despite the important benefits associated with the application of these concepts, there may be conflicts between economic health service delivery and concepts of schizophrenia respectful of the interpersonal aspects of illness. Linking service delivery systems together is important but may be harmful when it precludes the continuity of a therapeutic relationship. The patient needs an enduring relationship of this kind so that he is not faced with a stranger each time there is a significant change in clinical status.

Considering such lapses in continuity, it is not surprising that enormous numbers of schizophrenic patients fail to attend their first appointment in an aftercare clinic, and that others do not persevere. This is partly explained by apathy and other aspects of the illness, such as negativity or suspiciousness, but we believe that the unreasonable burden placed on a patient to establish (over and over) an interpersonal context for treatment contributes greatly to many of the problems in long-term treatment. In this regard, it is worth noting that there is an illusory cost effectiveness in providing services which can claim to be available to everyone, while unwittingly excluding the majority of people who require such care.

The concept of triage, while basically valuable when resources are in short supply, has often been used inappropriately in the treatment of schizophrenic patients. With such patients, triage processes wittingly or unwittingly applied have usually selected the more acute and better prognosis patients for higher quality care, while the chronic patients with poorer prognosis have often been assigned minimal treatment resources. But such triage, questionable on a humanitarian basis, may not even be optimal for therapeutic impact and resource utilization.

The tendency to select the good prognosis patients for maximum care may be based on faulty logic. What may appear to be successful early intervention preventing deterioration in the good prognosis patients may be only a reflection of a more benign natural course found in these patients in contrast to that of more chronic schizophrenia. It is possible that equal efforts with chronic patients could lead to an equal or greater improvement increment than they would with good prognosis patients, considering what otherwise would be their "natural course."[15] This possibility is supported by recent evidence showing that the potential range of outcome in chronic schizophrenia is far wider than was once believed. Some workers have described considerable symptomatic and social improvement in chronic patients after many years of deterioration. Most noteworthy are the studies by Manfred Bleuler[16] and Paul.[8]

Until we can base administrative decisions about who should receive the best care on sound evidence, we urge practicing clinicians to provide optimal treatment across the full prognostic range. Perhaps the course of disorder in more chronic patients would improve more if adequate resources were used.

There is also the question of how much of the available resources ought to be allocated for the treatment of schizophrenia generally. Society has not shown an appropriate concern for the effects of schizophrenia on its population; we have discussed this in more detail in Chapter 6. While easy to note, it appears that the mental health professions as well as society are years away from an appropriate advocacy of health care and research for this disorder. A quick reflection on the status of schizophrenia in society compared to, say, cancer, is sufficient to make this point. In the meantime, the clinician must struggle to provide the best possible care for patients in the absence of adquate resources and to provide rational clinical concepts upon which improved administrative decisions can be based.

SUMMARY

Since schizophrenia is a complex disorder, attention must be paid to several basic concepts in the planning and carrying out of treatment. These concepts include the establishment of a clear structure for patient assessment and treatment, the key role of ongoing personal involvement by the clinician during the treatment process, the interaction of interpersonal and psychopharmacological treatments, the collaboration of clinician and patient in treatment decisions, and attention to the various functional axes in treatment planning. These measures will lead to good care without necessarily lowering the cost of the care. More treatment resources for this disorder are urgently needed.

RECOMMENDED READING

Cancro, R., Fox, N., and Shapiro, L. E. (eds.). *Strategic intervention in schizophrenia*. New York: Behavioral Publications, 1974.

Gunderson, J. Individual psychotherapy. In: *Disorders of the schizophrenic syndrome*, Bellak, L. (ed.). New York: Basic Books, 1979, 364–398.

Lipton, M. A., and Burnett, G. B. Pharmacological treatment of schizophrenia. In: *Disorders of the schizophrenic syndrome*, Bellak, L. (Ed.). New York: Basic Books, 1979, 320–352.

Mendel, W. M. *Schizophrenia: The experience and its treatment*. San Francisco: Jossey–Bass, Inc., 1976.

Schulz, C. G., and Kilgalen, R. K. *Case studies in schizophrenia*. New York: Basic Books, 1969.

REFERENCES

1. Levy, S. T., McGlashan, T. H., and Carpenter, W. T., Jr. Integration and sealing-over as recovery styles from acute psychosis: Metapsychological and dynamic concepts. *Journal of Nervous and Mental Disease*, 1975, 161:307–312.
2. McGlashan, T. H., and Carpenter, W. T., Jr. Does attitude towards psychosis relate to outcome? *American Journal of Psychiatry*, in press.
3. Jackson, H. Remarks on evolution and dissolution of the nervous system. *Journal of Mental Science*, 1887, 33:25—48.
4. Strauss, J. S., Kokes, R. F., Ritzler, B. A., Harder, D. W., and VanOrd, A. Patterns of disorder in first admission psychiatric patients. *Journal of Nervous and Mental Disease*, 1978, 166(9):611–625.
5. Carpenter, W. T., Jr., and Heinrichs, D. W. Treatment of relevant subtypes of schizophrenia. *Journal of Nervous and Mental Disease*, in press.
6. Bachrach, L. L. Planning mental health services for chronic patients. *Hospital and Community Psychiatry*, 1979, 30:387–393.
7. Clausen, J. The impact of mental illness: A 20-year follow-up. In: *Life history research in psychopathology*, vol. 4, Wirt, R. D., Winokur, G., and Roff, M. (eds.). Minneapolis, MN: University of Minnesota Press, 1976, 270–289.
8. Paul, G. L. Comprehensive psychosocial treatment: Beyond traditional psychotherapy. In: *Psychotherapy of schizophrenia*, Strauss, J. S. *et al.* (eds.). New York: Plenum, 1980.
9. Liberman, R. P., Wallace, C. J., Vaughn, C. E., Snyder, K. S., and Rust, C. Social and family factors in the course of schizophrenia: Towards an interpersonal problem-solving therapy for schizophrenics and their families. In: *Psychotherapy of schizophrenia*, Strauss, J. S. *et al.* (eds.). New York: Plenum, 1980.
10. Anthony, W. Psychological rehabilitation: A concept in need of a method. *American Psychologist*, 1977, 658–662.
11. Carpenter, W. T., Jr., McGlashan, T. H., and Strauss, J. S. The treatment of acute schizophrenia without drugs: An investigation of some current assumptions. *American Journal of Psychiatry*, 1977, 134:14–20.
12. Wynne, L. C., Toohey, M. L., and Doane, J. Family studies. In: *Disorders of the schizophrenic syndrome*, Bellak, L. (ed.). New York: Basic Books, 1979, 264–288.
13. Leff, J. P. Schizophrenia and sensitivity to the family environment. *Schizophrenia Bulletin*, 1976, 2:566–574.
14. Scott, R. D. Closure in family relationships and the first official diagnosis. In: *Schizophrenia '75: Psychotherapy, family studies, research*, Jorstad, J., and Ugelstad, E. (eds.). Oslo: Universitetsforlaget, 1976, 265–281.
15. Strauss, J. S., and Frader, M. A. Justifying intensive psychotherapy for schizophrenia in a community treatment center. In: *Schizophrenia '75: Psychotherapy, family studies, research*, Jorstad, J. & Ugelstad, E. (eds.). Oslo: Universitetsforlaget, 1976.
16. Bleuler, M. The long-term course of the schizophrenic psychoses. *Psychological Medicine*, 1974, 4:244–254.

CHAPTER 10

Treatments

GUIDELINES AND MODALITIES

Treatment for schizophrenia has never been satisfactory, and this is still true today even though the clinician can now draw upon a number of available treatment methods. Nonetheless, very significant progress has been accomplished during the middle third of the twentieth Century, and the degree of hopelessness and therapeutic nihilism previously associated with the diagnosis of schizophrenia is no longer warranted.

Three major treatment developments have marked this recent period. The first of these has been the improvement of interpersonal therapeutic strategies derived from psychoanalytic theory and aimed at effecting psychological change in schizophrenic patients. While the therapeutic efficacy of such approaches is still debated, our understanding of the schizophrenic patient's subjective experiences and interpersonal pathology has been remarkably enhanced, and these therapeutic approaches have had a humanizing effect on the treatment of this illness.

The second major therapeutic development is an offshoot of social psychiatry. Brave innovations by hospital superintendents in England early in the 1950s have led to widespread administrative changes in the treatment of schizophrenic patients. Hospital wards are less likely to be locked, hospitals are less isolated, the base of hospital care has shifted toward the community, and treatment expectations now routinely include anticipation of discharge with the possibility of readmission, rather than lengthy, perhaps lifelong, institutional care. In this country, the community mental health center movement has increased the resources available for the treatment of discharged schizophrenic patients. Although still fraught with problems in making continuity of care available to the thousands of poverty-level schizophrenic individuals, these changes have created settings for treatment remarkably different from the custodial ambience which they succeeded.

The third major innovation has been the introduction of antipsychotic drugs. These medications have been used since the early 1950s and include numerous derivatives of four chemical classes. These drugs affect many neurophysiological systems, but all are similar in their inhibition of dopaminergic neuronal systems. In numerous studies, they have proven effective in reducing psychotic symptoms and in delaying or preventing psychotic relapse.

The availability of effective antipsychotic drugs is often used as the sole explanation for the incredible reduction in the number of hospitalized schizophrenics during the past 25 years. It seems more reasonable to view antipsychotic medication as providing an important (perhaps indispensable) contribution to the massive changes in treatment already initiated by the social psychiatry movement and to credit all three innovations mentioned above with providing a more humane and therapeutic approach to schizophrenic patients. The patient today spends less time in the hospital and is therefore less likely to become isolated from his community and the everyday expectations of life, and effective therapy aimed at reduction of psychotic symptoms is now available. These advances in treatment and the appreciation that various modalities are not mutually exclusive provide a wide range of possibilities for the therapy of schizophrenic patients, but most are nonspecific and none can be touted as curative. Before discussing specific treatment modalities in detail, we note three general guidelines for treatment planning implicit in the previous chapter.

First, treatment will vary tremendously from patient to patient and from circumstance to circumstance. The diagnosis of schizophrenia in itself is only a limited value for suggesting treatment, and thus, a cookbook approach to the treatment needs of schizophrenia is not feasible. For this reason, we will present key points related to treatment planning, realizing that specific decision-making must reside with the clinician working with the individual patient.

Second, the individualization of care is enhanced by the many modalities of treatment that can be given simultaneously or phased over time in various combinations. The resulting complexity should not discourage multimodality therapeutics.

Third, treatment and evaluation are intertwined. The process of relating and information exchange that begins with the first contact is an important part of both evaluation and treatment. Just as treatment may begin with the first contact, evaluation and the need to modify treatment accordingly continue throughout the treatment program.

SPECIFIC TREATMENT MODALITIES

Residential Treatment

Residential treatment modalities include a wide range of settings, but psychiatric hospitals and psychiatric units in general hospitals are the most common. Hospitals can and should be institutions that decrease morbidity and enhance adaptive functioning. A severely disturbed patient has much to gain from hospital-based care. Conferring the patient role can provide a structure which reduces ambiguity and decreases the level of provocative stimulation. Temporarily, the patient is relieved of the stress and burden of certain responsibilities. The hospital is a setting in which the interpersonal basis of diagnosis and treatment can be established. For these reasons, anxiety, perplexity, and other symptoms may diminish rapidly following admission to the hospital.

Hospitalization may also reduce the social and legal consequences of psychotic behavior. If the person behaves strangely at work, he may permanently impair his job and his work relationships. Bizarre behavior has obvious social and sometimes legal consequences that increase isolation and lower the expectations that society may have of the offending individual. Conferring the role of patient and removing the person from his ordinary social context can forestall expulsion from the work and social environments.

It is obvious that hospitals should be reserved for those in special need, but the current emphasis on avoiding hospitalization of the schizophrenic patient at all cost reveals a serious misunderstanding of the role of hospital care. The harmful effects of chronic hospitalization used for custodial purposes[1,2] should not conceal the very positive gains associated with therapeutic hospital care. A thousand days of hospital care may be far more negative than 100 days, but it does not then follow that 100 days are worse than 10 and 10 worse than 7 or none.

Negative Implications of Hospitalization

In spite of the value and necessity of hospital care, it is often seen by the patient, family, clinician, hospital staff, and community as evidence of personal or treatment failure. The view of hospitalization as failure is reflected strikingly in epidemiological studies and in research on treatment effectiveness. In both instances, rehospitalization is often the sole criterion of treatment failure or "recidivism"[3]—an ominous-sounding term, at best. This negative view of hospitalization may impede recovery and complicate posthospital adjustment; for example, families of patients repeatedly hospitalized tend to withdraw and look elsewhere for key emotional and instrumental relationships.[4]

Pessimistic views of hospitalization unduly complicate the therapeutic use of hospitals. The alternative has been to avoid or abbreviate hospitalization at all costs, and one cost is now observed to be large numbers of patients with vegetative existences living out a myth of community care. We think comprehensive care in the community is vital, but this must include (not exclude!) therapeutic hospitals. Admission to a hospital can signify that a patient has run into trouble in his attempt to lead a full life rather than accepting a more sheltered and incomplete existence.[5] Furthermore, schizophrenia is often a relapsing illness. Can one imagine treatment attitudes that denigrate therapeutic hospital care in other severe, relapsing illnesses (e.g., myocardial infarction)?

Duration of Hospitalization

Many factors determine the optimal length of hospital care,[6] and these factors vary from patient to patient and hospital to hospital. To establish an ideal length of stay and require justification for deviation belies the heterogeneity of the disease and of the social–medical circumstances. To say that long-term residential stay in custodial care has deleterious effects is not to deny that good alternatives exist for chronically disabled patients. Some patients require prolonged stay in a sheltered environment, others may benefit from long-term therapeutic hospital care, many others should receive briefer hospital-based treatment, and still others are better off when episodes of illness are treated outside the hospital. Are there principles other than asserting that duration of stay should be individualized? Yes.

1. Hospital care should be part of a larger treatment effort and

continuity of care provided by one, or at most two, primary clinicians continuously involved with the patient. This can reduce the duration of stay by providing diagnosis, evaluation, patient–clinician relationship, comprehensive treatment plan, informed consent, family participation, and social network assessment at the outset, thereby avoiding delays in treatment implementation.

2. Sufficient time should be provided to assure that the purpose of hospital care is understood. A clinician caring for a patient as he decompensates may have a good grasp of circumstances contributing to the patient's relapse, and can make a thoughtful judgment concerning discharge three days later as symptom reduction and impulse control are achieved. However, the same three-day hospital stay will be too brief for a clinician unfamiliar with the patient to accomplish the necessary evaluation and planning. The primary treatment opportunity may be removal of the patient from a chaotic environment which is precipitating a relapse. Discharge prior to attaining some improvement in environment or in the patient's ability to cope will have missed the therapeutic opportunity.

3. The clinician deciding whether to hospitalize a patient will consider negative and positive psychosocial consequences of the action. Similarly, decisions regarding discharge must take into account the consequences of reentering the non-hospital environment. Many factors must be balanced (e.g., difficulty in adjusting if prematurely discharged vs. losing one's job if absent too long); hence, hospital care should be of sufficient duration to permit informed judgments concerning the patient's environment and his ability to cope as well as his mental status.

4. The capacity of the hospital's therapeutic approach to be effective must be assessed in general and applied to each individual patient. A hospital organized extensively for crisis intervention and rapid return to the community may be poorly suited to undertake interpersonal therapies aimed at decreasing the patient's psychological vulnerability or enhancing familial support. Similarly, a therapeutic environment geared to an intermediate range of psychosocial goals may be ill prepared to treat and discharge a patient rapidly or to provide long-term sheltering. When a hospital is unable to offer the full range of care opportunities, the clinician must take this into account in decisions on the duration of stay. However, rather than attempting to fit every patient into the hospital's philosophy, the clinician should consider what is optimal for the patient and select a therapeutic environment suited to these needs.

5. Hospital care should include discharge planning, reintegration

into a non-hospital environment, arrangements for continuity of care, and provisions for follow-up. Neither the planning nor implementation can be accomplished quickly unless continuity of clinicians providing care is already in place. Time is needed, and pressures that force patients out of hospitals before they or their families are prepared run the risk of treatment neglecting crucial clinical considerations. Patients often experience the care system as so impersonal that little motivation is provided for participation in outpatient treatment.

No matter how long the hospitalization, it is important that the clinician, and usually the patient, keep in contact with appropriate family members. Often these people have basic unanswered questions, feel left out, worried, and uncertain.[7] Often, too, because of physical distance and limited resources, the medical system focuses on the patient alone, ignoring his or her social ties, and, because it is "simpler," may actively exclude family to the ultimate detriment of the patient, who will be returning to that environment. This problem has been aggravated recently by insurance regulations prohibiting coverage for patients spending days or weekends out of the hospital, even when this is judged indispensable to maintaining community ties.

Thus, hospitalization may serve many treatment purposes. It should always provide an opportunity for evaluation and reevaluation of the patient, including fundamental aspects of diagnosis and conceptualization of treatment needs. It is good that the day when a schizophrenic patient was hospitalized and "the key was thrown away" has passed. It will not be satisfying to the intelligent clinician to substitute for these old stereotypes new, rigid rules which require minimal use of hospitalization and arbitrary limits on stay, rather than an acknowledgment of the variability in needs and the necessity for clinical judgment incorporating a broad range of relevant data. There is a confluence of data from several studies suggesting that many patients find hospital programs providing multifactorial treatment lasting 30–100 days to be optimal.[8] Today's hospitals tend toward less than 30 days or more than 6 months.

Partial Hospitalization and Related Treatment

An extremely important group of treatment facilities has become increasingly available in recent years. These include a variety of partial hospitalization, halfway house, and other residential therapeutic settings which increase the clinician's capacity to achieve an optimal balance between risks and benefits associated with residential treatment and community living. These treatment facilities will not be discussed in detail here. In general, the principles governing their applicability are implied in the comments on hospitalization and other specific therapeutic modalities and the general principles and guidelines for treatment. The use of these facilities is determined by their availability—or, more commonly, by their unavailability. The shortage of intermediate care facilities forces arbitrary decisions between total hospitalization and nonresidential care. This unfortunate situation is costly and makes discharge planning particularly difficult and the process of return to the community a period of stress.

Individual Psychotherapy

In discussing this disputed topic, we shall describe some of the controversies involved and our interpretation of them and then suggest some guidelines for traversing these troubled waters until clinical research provides a firmer basis for reaching conclusions.

Since the concept of schizophrenia was established, most workers in most settings have presumed psychotherapy irrelevant. The roots for this assumption can be identified in Freud's statement that the schizophrenic patient cannot form a transference relationship and also in Jaspers' belief that the schizophrenic patient cannot establish empathic bonds which permit another person to understand his schizophrenic experiences. The result has been that most psychiatrists interested in psychodynamic treatments have not been interested in schizophrenia, and many psychiatrists interested in description of psychopathology have been disinterested in understanding the subjective experiences of the schizophrenic patient.[9]

Nonetheless, a significant impact has been generated by clinicians who subscribe to interpersonal theories and treatment of schizophrenia. Much of this impact originated in the United States, arising especially during the heyday of psychodynamic psychiatry. At that time, interpersonal approaches to schizophrenia were generally accepted so long as specific treatments were not available. Later, the introduction of antipsychotic drugs set the stage for the drugs versus psychotherapy controversy, and a critical assessment of psychotherapeutic approaches.

These efforts involved a small number of important studies of psychotherapy for schizophrenia, generally with methodologies suitable for testing drug effects, but less appropriate for testing the efficacy of individual psychotherapy.[10] These studies usually led to the conclusion that drugs were therapeutically efficacious for schizophrenia, while psychotherapy was not. The first conclusion is valid, but the second has not yet received adequate scrutiny. This research and its conclusions have been criticized by psychotherapists, but proponents of interpersonal therapeutics have generally failed to take seriously the task of conducting well designed investigations to correct the methodological failings they have criticized.

Studying psychotherapy of schizophrenia does present many complex issues, and it is difficult to resolve key methodological problems. Nonetheless, the effort to do so is late, and today's clinician must determine the role of psychotherapy in each case, using experience, intuition, and treatment philosophy without benefit of a solid base of scientific knowledge.

Some argue that psychotherapy should be offered to schizophrenics only after satisfactory demonstration of efficacy, but we think this conclusion is unwarranted for two reasons. First, it assumes that the negative studies of psychotherapeutic efficacy are methodologically adequate, an assumption we believe is not justified from our review of such studies. Second, schizophrenic patients have crucial problems in the sphere of interpersonal relationships and intrapsychic functioning. While we are uncertain about the extent to which psychotherapeutic efforts will cause beneficial readjustment, alternative therapeutic tools with established efficacy are not available. Thus, it is sensible to attempt to establish a therapeutic relationship with a patient who has difficulty relating, to use this relationship to explore aspects of the patient's inner world where bewilderment and mystery impede recovery, and to provide a model for identification to patients with fluid and destructive self-concepts.

SOME GUIDELINES FOR PSYCHOTHERAPY OF SCHIZOPHRENIC PATIENTS

Reality Issues

As a schizophrenic patient relates his experiences, his primary process communications, mystification, and symbolic speech may enthrall both patient and therapist. The clinician is surely interested in these experiences, and their exploration may provide a basis for establishing a relationship with some patients, but exclusive attention to such phenomena is ill-advised. Excessive focus on these experiences has the risk of reinforcing dominating fantasies or provoking regression. Furthermore, if the therapist fails also to explore the patient's functioning in ordinary areas such as work, social relationships, participation in other aspects of the treatment program, and family relations, then patient and clinician will be oblivious to many of the key manifestations of illness, and the patient's strengths and areas of competence will not receive appropriate recognition. The therapist's inquiry into ordinary life functioning helps to clarify his expectations of the patient and will provide a more suitable model for identification. Finally, considerable focus on reality will keep the patient and therapist more closely attuned to the major goals of treatment and will help make that treatment more understandable to other mental health workers and to the family.

But a focus on reality does not exclude attention to issues of meaning and fantasy. The therapist of a schizophrenic patient must "work both sides of the street," in continually examining the juxtaposition of reality and feelings and psychotic distortions. If a goal of psychotherapy is to reduce vulnerability to stressful factors, it is obvious that the therapist must strive toward both the identification of stressors and the understanding of the patient's reactions to them.

A clinical vignette will illustrate this point. During outpatient psychotherapy, a patient began bringing his art for discussion. The art work was intriguing and the patient's remarks and associations were highly informative concerning intrapsychic conflict and symptom formation. With attention focused on the paintings rather than on the person, the patient was able to explore his experiences with less anxiety. But the preoccupation with artistic production in and out of sessions decreased the patient's ties to reality, and, without anxiety as a check against regression, the patient's cognitive disorganization reappeared.

At first, this was interpreted as a defense against the intrapsychic conflict being examined through the art work. However, the patient's parents requested an urgent meeting to say that they had become quite concerned with changes taking place in the patient's behavior. Exploration of the basis for their concern revealed that the patient was staying up nights alone in his room, had begun sleeping late in the morning, attended no meals with his family, and did not have any social contact outside the home. His job-seeking activity had ceased, and he became quickly irritable with any demands to perform routine household tasks.

This and related information about the real situation suggested also that the cognitive disorganization was associated with increasing demands and anger on the part of the family and with the patient's withdrawal from social functioning. With this data, the therapist was able to redirect attention to the ordinary functioning of the patient, while maintaining (but limiting) an interest in the art works and the psychological explorations around them. Temporary reinstitution of antipsychotic medication proved useful, as did a family session which encouraged the parents to interfere with the patient's withdrawal into fantasy and to maintain a steady expectation of work performance at home, interpersonal contacts with the family, and the spending of some time away from home pursuing work and social opportunities.

The Relationship

Central to psychotherapy with schizophrenic patients is the relationship with the therapist, including its value in the process of identification and the reduction of isolation. The concept of the psychotherapist as a relatively inactive, neutral figure serving as a mirror of the patient's unconscious is not a tenable model for therapeutic work with schizophrenic patients. Many schizophrenic patients have an impaired capacity to understand another person; hence, the therapist's clarifications of his or her needs can be insight-inducing, and distortions destructive to therapy may be curtailed. Moreover, most psychotherapeutic techniques involve, wittingly or not, a process whereby the patient becomes more like the therapist. Although psychoanalytic work with neurotic patients requires the maintenance of a degree of ambiguity concerning the therapist, the psychotic patient is well served by the therapist's more actively but nonintrusively facilitating the process of identification. This may be an effective inducement to change and also assists the patient in recognizing similarities between himself and others which can be enormously reassuring.

The psychotherapist for schizophrenic patients is a participant/ observer involved in the therapeutic relationship in a manner that permits identification while keeping clear boundaries, facilitates acknowledgement of similarities and differences, and provides an opportunity for the patient to reduce the burden of privacy concerning perplexing subjective experiences.

Insight

Another mainstay of psychotherapeutic technique is the development of insight. While insight often implies an understanding of one's own intrapsychic conflicts, we would broaden the meaning in working with schizophrenic patients to include the developing of a rational and understandable framework for conceptualizing the personal imprint of psychotic experiences. Furthermore, it should include an appreciation of sequential relationships between environmental factors and symptom development. Pursuit of this task requires an exploration of positive symptoms such as delusions and hallucinations, an appreciation of their symbolic meaning, and a comprehension of the personal meaning of psychotic experiences more generally.

One further value of insight-oriented psychotherapy with schizophrenic patients is its use for clarifying the extent to which psychotic symptoms are gratifying. Psychotic patients are often in anguish, but clinicians may fail to notice those aspects of the experience that may be reassuring or gratifying. Such positive aspects take many forms, but the sense of power from impulsivity, the enthrallment with perplexity, the smugness of the grandiose, the comforting organization of delusions, the companionship provided by hallucinations, the excitement of suspiciousness, and the importance of the self-referential must be discerned and taken into account with all the various treatment modalities used. This aspect of illness can obviously be antitherapeutic, and there are many instances in which patients have withdrawn from somatic and psychological treatments which threatened to reduce gratifications associated with psychotic experience.

Clinicians may be hesitant to explore the meanings of symptoms with the patient during active psychosis, fearing that symptomatology may worsen or that the patient cannot benefit from understanding and insight. Later, many clinicians hesitate to examine symptomatology and the personal meaning of psychosis for fear that there will be a reawakening of such experiences or that the patient will be uncomfortable. We argue the converse; that is, during psychotic experiences the patients have no choice but to be confronted with bizarre thoughts, percepts, and ideation. The important question is whether there will be an opportunity to share these experiences with another individual or whether the patient must face them alone. Most friends, spouses, parents, and acquaintances discourage the patient from communicating these experiences to them.

The clinician has a different frame of reference and can provide the one opportunity for the patient to relieve himself of the burden of privacy without fear of the societal consequences. We know of no convincing data that exploration of such experiences causes them to worsen. Rather, we believe that systematically discouraging a patient from talking about psychotic experiences creates the illusion that the patient is less disturbed than he is while reinforcing psychological isolation.

The argument for exploration after psychotic symptomatology has subsided is even more straightforward. Some degree of insight into illness is required to achieve the patient's cooperation in any aspect of the treatment program. Any person passing through a chaotic and threatening personal crisis will have an innate need for psychological reconciliation. The clinician has a vested interest in the nature of closure achieved by the patient. To deprive the patient of the opportunity to use the clinician's perspective on the cause, meaning, and consequence of the illness is to invite idiosyncratic and destructive psychological closure.

We believe the key issue is an understanding of a person's needs once the fabric of life is torn asunder by psychosis. It is a mistake to mandate insight-oriented exploration on the basis of therapeutic ambition (for we do not yet know how therapeutic this approach is, or for whom) or etiological theory (for the etiology is uncertain). Furthermore, patients differ tremendously in their interests and their ability to profit from insight-oriented therapy, and a judgment will be required in determining which patients this approach to psychotherapy will benefit most decisively over an extended period of time. What may wisely be provided for all patients is the opportunity, to the extent that it is useful, to share their psychotic experience with a clinician, to develop a framework for understanding the personal significance, timing, and implications of their illness, and to reach a resolution of crisis with as little distortion and mystery as is feasible.

Affectivity and Negative Symptoms

The affectivity of the schizophrenic patient[11] requires special consideration by the psychotherapist. Ordinarily, a patient's affect is informative about the importance and meaning of experiences being reported and may function as a signal. However, affective lability, blunting, and displacement in schizophrenic patients can readily mislead the clinician in assessing the importance of the material under consideration, and motivation for psychological exploration is diminished. Nonetheless, specific consideration of these issues may provide the patient with an understanding of his effect on other people and his difficulty in perceiving and weighing the communications and intentions of others. Dealing with negative symptoms such as apathy and blunted affect is difficult, but the patient may find the clinician's observations (e.g., "Your problems in feeling enthusiastic with other people may trouble them as well as you") a useful orientation. Nonverbal activities are often necessary with the apathetic and withdrawn patient. Walking together, sharing coffee, etc., can serve as a basis for slowly increasing trust between the patient and the clinician and also for reducing some of the pressure to interact verbally. Such pressure frequently appears to have a discouraging impact on the patient's self-esteem and will prove frustrating to the therapist as well.

To the extent that blunting of affect is an effort to cope with cognitive or personality disorganization, the psychotherapist may intervene by seeking alternatives to prevent disorganization, such as reducing stresses, resolving intrapsychic conflict, using antipsychotic medication, helping the patient change his living environment, or periodic use of hospitalization. The blunting of affect is a phenomenon for which continued evaluation is crucial since this sign may have so many origins: it may arise as a primary negative symptom of schizophrenia, as a fear of social contacts, as secondary to postpsychotic depression, or it may be associated with akinesia and drug-induced apathy.

When apathy, negativism, lack of spontaneity and initiative, failure of affective arousal, and loss of reinforcing gratification are present, it is difficult indeed for the therapist to maintain the treatment task. Therefore, the psychotherapist working with the schizophrenic patient must be prepared to identify these processes and explore them to the extent possible. The exploration may reveal whether or not they can be influenced by psychotherapeutic techniques and whether they can be accounted for by other aspects of the patient's condition that might be changed. For example, with the long-term medicated patient, a period without drugs would clarify the extent to which negative symptoms were drug-induced side effects, an interaction between illness and drug effects, or unrelated to current medication.

As with any treatment approach, the psychotherapist must acknowledge the necessity for change in treatment when certain attributes of illness may best be treated by, or in conjunction with, other techniques. In respect to negative symptoms, programs using behavioral paradigms and learning techniques for altering behavior appear to be particularly promising, and social skills training procedures may enable the patient to reduce the complicating effects of prolonged social isolation and nonperformance in social and occupational tasks.

Dysphoric Symptoms

Harry Stack Sullivan reminded us that schizophrenic patients are more simply human than anything else. Too often, the less dramatic components of illness are ignored or regarded as unsuitable for psychotherapeutic intervention. We see no reason for the psychotherapist to judge the less florid symptoms in schizophrenic patients, such as depression, anxiety, or obsessions, as either not inviting treatment or unmodifiable with psychotherapeutic techniques. Unfortunately, these more ordinary aspects of illness may go unnoticed when they coexist with psychotic or negative symptoms. [12]

There are circumstances in which therapeutic modalities other than psychotherapy might be used for the nonpsychotic symptoms that occur in schizophrenia, but the clinician may be hesitant because of the patient's diagnosis. If a schizophrenic patient has a depressed episode of sufficient severity to require treatment, the therapist should consider the possible use of antidepressant medication. Caution should be based on the possible psychosis-inducing consequence of the pharmacotherapy, rather than on the assumptions that schizophrenic patients cannot become depressed or that depression in schizophrenia requires no special treatment.

Feelings and Attitudes of the Therapist

The clinician intimately involved in the process of treating schizophrenic patients, especially chronic patients, will often experience frustration, therapeutic nihilism, and despair regardless of what therapeutic modalities are utilized. Prognosis is variable but guarded, and we have no treatment strategy that can promise a cure. Therefore, the clinician needs to face his own feelings of doubt and hopelessness in order to preclude precipitous changes in therapeutic techniques unconsciously designed to relieve his own disquietude.

Some therapists are unjustifiably confident of the efficacy of their treatment, but the opposite problem is more frequent in clinicians treating schizophrenic patients. There can be a sense of no progress even in the face of significant benefit. This may be explained by the fact that psychopathological impairment in rapport, affect, or sense of self may be obvious in psychotherapy sessions even though work and relationships outside have improved. We have often been surprised by a patient's account of his accomplishments, finding ourselves preoccupied with the persevering impairments rather than with the new strengths.

Another cause of frustration is the setting of unrealistically high goals or providing insufficient time to accomplish goals. Aims of psychosocial interventions are usually long-term (e.g., increasing capacity for intimacy, reconciliation of intrapsychic conflict), but treatment milestones often have a shorter phase influenced by the striking episodes and remissions of psychosis.

Another source of difficulty is the clinician's (and often the patient's) feeling of defeat when a psychotic episode occurs following what was regarded as some degree of improvement. Here the clinician (and others) may misinterpret the meaning of psychotic decompensation and either attribute the psychosis to the treatment itself or assume that the psychotic episode is evidence against any therapeutic effect. It is important to appreciate the fact that the slow work of helping a patient find himself and establish a meaningful niche in society can coexist with an episodic course of illness. Although psychotherapy may reduce vulnerability to psychotic episodes, pharmacotherapy has more proven merit in this regard, and psychological treatment appears to be better suited for approaching intrapsychic and interpersonal manifestations of illness.

The personal frustrations for the clinician seem greater when the degree of involvement is greater. Hence, a patient who decompensates on maintenance antipsychotic medication is not likely to be faced with a clinician who gives up in despair and resolves that further drug therapy is unwarranted. But the patient's psychotherapist may well throw up his hands in despair, feeling somehow responsible for the psychotic episodes and incapable of providing further help to the patient. In this regard, we urge the clinician to keep in mind the complex interactive developmental model of illness that we set forth earlier. To date, treatment (any treatment) is only one of many contributors to the course of illness. No treatment can stand the test of preventing all future difficulties or benefitting all aspects of illness. The clinician must enable the patient, family, and himself to maintain that perspective.

One final caveat on attitude. The psychotherapy of schizophrenia need not be based on etiological theory. The therapist who assumes that all aspects of schizophrenia are caused by personally meaningful connections will mislead and ultimately frustrate the patient and himself. We urge the clinician to help the patient gain some personal perspective, for example, on the content of his delusions without implying that this will explain the occurrence of that particular type of symptom. A patient can understand why familial tensions are so distressing without assuming that these tensions have *caused* schizophrenia. The polemics associated with competing etiological theories should not undermine the practical approach of the clinician to the patient in a disorganizing personal crisis.

Repetition, Reporting, and Boredom

On occasion, psychotherapy sessions may be dull, marked by bland reporting of events and repetition of previous statements and problems without any progress. Therapists may hesitate to comment to the patient about such instances, as though to do so would be futile or provocative. Such hesitation may reflect the common belief that schizophrenic patients are so fragile that clinicians must use extreme caution in any interactions. But excessive restraint creates a confusing and dehumanizing process which only serves further to isolate the patient. The therapist, gently but firmly, must pursue such problems in the therapeutic process with the patient. Pointed observations can be helpful, such as, "You often raise this issue, but you show little emotion about it and nothing changes." The difficult but essential process of pursuing such points while attempting to maximize tact and good timing must then ensue. Blocks to therapeutic progress must be confronted and explored with schizophrenic patients just as with others.

Consultation and Supervision

Because the psychotherapy of schizophrenia is bewildering and the clinician needs to integrate psychotherapy into a multifactorial treatment approach, supervision and consultation are frequently needed. The use of a consultant at points of crisis, despair, or the therapist's loss of a shared set of expectations with the patient or the patient's family can be illuminating. It can relieve the psychotherapist from bearing the sole professional burden for evaluating treatment alternatives, and it can provide the family and/or the patient with a perspective of a clinician not deeply enmeshed in the interpersonal aspects of therapy. If trees obscure the forest, consultation provides a good chance of regaining perspective. In those instances when patient and therapist have reached such loggerheads that it is not possible for them to continue, the consultant can help both to achieve a constructive separation from the treatment effort.

Consultations generally seem to work best if: (1) the consultant feels free to consider all aspects of treatment; (2) it is clear beforehand to whom he will give his report (patient, clinician, family, any two, or all three); (3) the clinician feels free to take or reject the advice; and (4) the patient is free to find a new clinician if a specific incompatibility between the patient and clinician exists that cannot be resolved. These simple guidelines can make what could be an interpersonally confusing process clear and helpful.

For the clinician with limited experience in working with schizophrenic patients, supervision is vitally important. Even for the most experienced therapist, the bizarre and alienating aspects of the psychopathology may cause intense transference and countertransference problems. The difficulty of using psychotherapy with schizophrenic patients can be further complicated if, as often happens, there is not a supportive milieu within which this enterprise can be undertaken. Clinicians who are encouraged to have a professional identity as entirely self-sufficient are surprised by how meaningful the support of a colleague can be in pursuing this difficult task.

Psychological Strengths

Despite the severity and urgency of many problems in schizophrenia, it is crucial that patient and therapist not focus solely on psychopathological manifestations. Identifying areas of strength can have a valuable effect on the patient; the therapist acknowledges the successful and effective aspects of the patient's behavior, thereby encouraging maximum utilization of these strengths to reduce the patient's tendency to incorporate them into areas of pathological functioning. The long-term follow-up studies in Switzerland lend support to this emphasis, noting that successful outcome is associated with treatment involving a continuous relationship with a clinician who can relate to the patient's strengths.[13,14] Still more recently, exploratory research has been carried on to establish a model for combining treatment focus on both strengths and problems.[15]

OTHER PSYCHOSOCIAL MODALITIES

There are a number of other interpersonal therapeutic techniques potentially beneficial to the schizophrenic patient. Many issues discussed in relation to dyadic psychotherapy also apply to these other strategies and, therefore, will be discussed only briefly here.

Group Therapy

Since schizophrenic patients have profound difficulties in establishing and maintaining social ties, group therapy is a treatment modality that is particularly relevant to this disorder. Some, but not all, schizophrenic patients will find evocative, exploratory groups too stimulating or expectations too high, but in many therapeutic groups, interpersonal pressures are often lower than those associated with clinician–patient and other dyadic relationships.

There is evidence that certain forms of group therapy are particularly useful for schizophrenic patients.[8,16] It appears to be especially helpful if focused primarily on concrete problems of relating and function and only secondarily on achieving insight. Some forms of group treatment, such as social clubs and activity groups, offer socialization experiences without a psychotherapeutic philosophy. The aim here is to learn and practice basic social skills and to share a sense of purpose with other people.

Conjoint Family Therapy

To what extent should the family be involved in the treatment of a schizophrenic patient? Frequently the need may be considerable. To begin with, the family is an important source of information on the patient's milieu and on other key data necessary in diagnosis and treatment. Besides this, family members need help from clinicians in understanding schizophrenia and knowing what it involves, what causes it, and what to expect. Most important of all, they frequently need guidance regarding their fears, the goals of treatment, and how they should deal with the patient.[7]

In several instances, family interaction patterns may contribute to the disorder and its course. There is good evidence suggesting that intrusive or excessively hostile family relationships are associated with recurrence of symptoms in the schizophrenic person.[17] Clinical observation also has long suggested that other types of interaction between family members and the schizophrenic patient may have a destructive effect on some or all of the individuals involved.

Although research on family treatment has been both relatively rare and controversial, some evidence for efficacy has been generated.[18] Recent findings suggest that family therapy and drug therapy have a particularly beneficial interaction.[19]

Considered together, these kinds of experience and evidence suggest the necessity of routinely involving family (or household) members in the clinical care of schizophrenic patients. Five major purposes for this involvement are particularly important: (a) to collect relevant data regarding the patient and his environment; (b) to assess the impact of illness on the family and determine what assistance they need; (c) to educate the family to provide a helpful milieu and to prevent premature extrusion of the patient from treatment; (d) to determine specific family/ illness interactions; and (e) to determine which families would profit from family therapy.

Behavior Therapy

Psychiatrists in particular have remained underinformed concerning the therapeutic potential of a variety of interpersonal approaches based on learning or conditioning paradigms. Paul[20] has reported many important benefits from behavioral techniques applied in cases of chronic patients for whom other treatments have failed. The application of social skills training and reinforcement techniques in the context of family therapy and individual sessions has also been described.[21] The potential to induce change with behavioral techniques is established, but further work is required to determine whether effects are generalizable (i.e., improvement in one skill may not result in improvement in other skills) and enduring. The interested reader is referred to recent reviews for a full description of techniques and philosophy.[22]

Other Modalities

There are other crucial interpersonal approaches to the treatment of schizophrenia which are not discussed here, partly because they fall somewhat outside our emphasis on the clinician–patient relationship. Of special importance are certain practical and often indispensable interventions such as social case work, occupational counseling, and vocational rehabilitation. The provision of fundamental support in living (e.g., rooming, income) is also often at issue,[18] and confusion abounds in any discussion of whether this should be considered clinical care or human services. In the context of this book, it is particularly important to state that these functional and environmental considerations are essential as part of the developmental interactive model of schizophrenia, and clinicians responsible for planning and conducting multifaceted treatment need to be competent in integrating these services into an overall therapeutic strategy. When these issues are at the forefront of a patient's life, they cannot be simply background for "treatment."

PSYCHOPHARMACOTHERAPY

The discussion of psychosocial modalities precedes that of somatic treatments because interpersonal strategies are the necessary foundation for treating schizophrenic patients. However, in discussing psychosocial treatments, we have complained about the lack of methodologically sound clinical investigations. In developing the psychosocial aspects of a treatment plan, the clinician is thus left with much of the responsibility for integrating experiences, available theory, anecdotal reports, and systematic research findings into a coherent treatment. In contrast, the field of pharmacology has made great strides in establishing the therapeutic efficacy and optimal regimens for using antipsychotic drugs to treat schizophrenic patients.

The reader will have noted a plaintive tone in our discussions of the way in which these drugs are used and the stress on pharmacotherapy that has been associated with a deemphasis of other aspects of treatment. In this section, we will describe briefly the rationale for using antipsychotic drugs and then provide some guidelines that will encourage the clinician to be prudent in pharmacotherapy. In doing so, we want to remind the reader that the introduction of antipsychotic drugs into the psychiatrist's armamentarium has been a major step forward in the treatment of schizophrenia and in providing a pathway toward understanding the biochemistry of schizophrenia. Whatever the limitations of pharmacotherapy, its contributions to clinical care and to the heuristics of scientific psychiatry have been enormous. The discussion is short because efficacy data and discussions of pharmacotherapy are well known and readily available.[22]

During the acute phases of psychosis, antipsychotic medications appear to have a significant effect on a broad range of psychopathology, including positive psychotic symptoms and behavioral and cognitive dysfunction. For example, anxiety is diminished (the calming effect led to the misnomer "major tranquilizer" during the 1950s). Delusions and hallucinations also respond to these agents. Formal thought disorder with disorganization and blocking of speech, which some workers view as the core deficiency in schizophrenia, shows a therapeutic response to these drugs, but apparently in a slower time frame than do delusions, hallucinations, and anxiety. Because aspects of panic, violence, impulsivity, belligerence, agitation, and pressured behavior are responsive to antipsychotic medication, these drugs become crucial to management of psychiatric emergencies in schizophrenic and nonschizophrenic patients.

The second well established and profoundly important clinical effect of antipsychotic medication is the capacity to reduce psychotic relapse and hospital readmission rates during aftercare. Patients successfully treated with medication during hospitalization can reduce their vulnerability to relapse about twofold if maintained on medication following discharge. This effect lasts at least four years, and one may surmise that it is a likely effect so long as a patient is in an episodic phase of illness.

A third potential, but unproven, therapeutic effect of antipsychotic medication is on deficit functioning or negative symptoms. These problems have not been thoroughly investigated, and the clinician has little research data from which to estimate the extent to which therapeutic leverage can be gained in these areas of function. The clinician must also weigh the possibility of a negative interaction between drug effects and illness effects on psychopathological attributes such as apathy, loss of spontaneity, and social dysfunction.

A fourth area of potential drug benefit is in the facilitation of psychosocial therapeutic techniques. This issue was long bogged down in nonproductive controversy, but clinicians are now less willing to conceptualize the two treatment approaches as mutually exclusive. Recent reports have demonstrated that the therapeutic benefit of psychosocial treatment is often enhanced by concomitant use of antipsychotic medication and vice versa.[19,23]

Limitations and Other Considerations
in Pharmacotherapy

1. The clinician should be mindful that no treatment specific for schizophrenia has been discovered. The antipsychotic drugs are not antischizophrenic in any strict sense. On the one hand, they have a broad range of application and are effective in conditions known, or thought, to have different etiologies (e.g., mania, psychotic features of organic psychosyndromes, brief reactive psychoses). On the other hand, there are important aspects of schizophrenic dysfunction for which these agents have no demonstrated efficacy. Thus, schizophrenic patients should not be treated as though they had "phenothiazine deficiency syndromes." Rather, in considering pharmacotherapy, attention should be focused on those specific phases of illness and psychopathological attributes for which these drugs are known to have beneficial effect.

2. We do not presently have a diversity of pharmacological approaches to schizophrenia. In patients who prove nonresponsive to antipsychotic medication, there is no alternative worth trying in the same sense that an MOA inhibitor may be useful in a depressive disorder which does not respond to tricyclic antidepressants. There is, however, every reason to believe that at least some drug nonresponders do not have adequate quantities of the drug available at physiological sites in the brain necessary for antipsychotic activity. There are presently no readily available techniques for differentiating between those nonresponders in whom idiosyncratic pharmacokinetics preclude adequate drug concentration at brain sites and those who do not respond despite adequate concentration of drugs in the appropriate areas. Plasma drug levels, where available, may guide the clinician in choosing some nonresponders for therapeutic trials at dose levels above the usual clinical practice.

3. In urgent treatment situations, an important problem arises if a therapeutic alliance has not been previously developed. Antipsychotic drugs have a profound effect on the patient's affect, behavior, and subjective experiences. A schizophrenic person may not understand our intentions, and suspiciousness is commonplace. Hence, an important clinical dilemma arises when the patient is subjected to the powerful effect of drugs without a context for understanding the therapeutic use of these medications. Sometimes this is unavoidable, and it may be essential to initiate treatment despite misunderstanding. However, we believe that

this problem is magnified when clinicians assume that the patient cannot cooperate or understand treatment considerations until psychotic symptoms remit. As psychotic distortions are reduced, greater clarification can be achieved; but it is a mistake to wait until that point to initiate a collaborative process. The fact that in emergency circumstances one may have to medicate a patient without his consent does not relieve us of the responsibility of maximizing the collaboration with the patient around acute pharmacotherapy. Patients often recall the details of discussions which took place when they were psychotic, even if they appeared inattentive at the time. In any case, it is important for clinicians to maintain the integrity of the collaboration and to discuss the treatment rationale with the patient even when the patient is unable to participate coherently.

4. There are several early side effects of antipsychotic medication which, when added to other treatment experiences, may seriously impair later treatment cooperation. Although usually neither dangerous nor lasting, the side effects can have an unsettling impact on a patient already bewildered by his experiences. The "noncompliance" that is so often a significant problem associated with the pharmacotherapy of schizophrenia may be intensified by these effects. While all physicians face the problem of patients' not adhering to therapeutic regimes, we cannot think of another situation in which noncompliance is so blatantly widespread and so poorly understood. Patients throw their medicines away during the acute phases of treatment, reduce their doses or discontinue medication following partial remission, leave hospitals covertly planning to discontinue their medication, and avoid outpatient appointments in order to avoid medication during aftercare.

The problem of side effects, when added to the other treatment problems in schizophrenia, further emphasizes the importance of establishing a therapeutic alliance for using medication in a context which maximizes the patient's understanding and minimizes suspiciousness and distortions. Sensitivity to the apprehension and discomforts associated with side effects, to the fear that another person might be able to induce powerful psychological effects, and to concerns about the obliteration of sometimes gratifying experiences is required. In many instances, the manner of using drugs seems to be "strike three" in the dehumanizing process. While the desired therapeutic end may be humanizing, patients with an illness replete with experiences that separate them from

other humans are met with clinical care situations where they are assumed unable to participate in their own treatment, often lose their
personal clothing and other belongings, have other people assuming
responsibility for ordinary functions of life, and are then provided with
medication which radically alters highly personal experiences. At times,
patients use whatever spirit remains to resist the efforts which we view as
therapeutically sound and which they may experience as dehumanizing.

5. Confusing or adverse drug–illness interactions may occur. Some
common side effects are difficult to distinguish from illness effects and
may complicate the course of illness. Akinesia, sedation, and a state of
apathetic depression can be associated with antipsychotic medication.
Similar effects have long been observed in the postpsychotic and the
chronic phases of schizophrenic illness. As illness effects, these are difficult phenomena to treat, but as drug side effects, they can be reversed.
Drug reduction, drug discontinuation, the addition of anti-Parkinsonian
medication, patient education concerning side effects, or switching to
another antipsychotic drug with a different side effect profile are possibilities.

Another drug complication sometimes misinterpreted as illness
manifestation is an anticholinergic crisis. Psychotic symptoms and confusion are associated with anticholinergic-induced organic psychosyndromes and in the schizophrenic patient may be mistaken for disease
exacerbation. Immediate and effective treatment (physostigmine, drug
discontinuation) is available. If the clinician mistakenly assumes the
increased symptomatology to be an exacerbation of schizophrenia, the
result will be to increase medications and the pharmacologically induced
anticholinergic activity. Delirium and peripheral anticholinergic effects
(e.g., bladder distention) are keys to differential diagnosis.

Multiple drug–drug interactions can occur when antipsychotic medication is given with other psychoactive drugs. Patients simultaneously
receiving an antidepressant, an antipsychotic, and an antiParkinsonian
drug are receiving three anticholinergic medications. Unpredictable
drug–drug interactions are one reason the clinician attempts to avoid
immediate use of antipsychotic medication when psychosis is induced
with impure street drugs. Antipsychotic drugs affect several neurotransmitter systems, and interactions with many drugs used in a variety
of medical conditions must be expected.

6. Many long-term adverse side effects of antipsychotic drugs have
been reported. Although some of these effects remain to be proven, a

general concern is warranted since the drugs profoundly affect so many systems. Effects such as reduction of motivation or spontaneity may never be discerned, since the illness is already known to be associated with personality deterioration. So-called secondary effects such as the impact of drugs on parenting behavior and consequently on the child's development will also elude discovery, since illness also affects parenting. Other general concerns such as carcinogenesis (breast tumors in mice and increased prolactic secretion in humans) have not been confirmed.

Because of their many effects, antipsychotic medications should not be used in pregnant women, except in dire circumstances, since these drugs cross the placental barrier and may alter neuronal development in the fetus as well as hormonal systems subserving reproductive functioning.

In spite of these concerns, the broad range of fears regarding the long-term side effects of antipsychotic drugs has not materialized into proven facts. In the short run, these drugs appear exceptionally safe, and most long-term concerns are balanced by known benefits. There is a major exception however: a late-onset drug-induced abnormal involuntary movement disorder called tardive dyskinesia.

Tardive dyskinesia[24-26] is the most important of the common neurological complications of antipsychotic drugs and threatens to alter profoundly the clinical use of these medications. Despite this syndrome's having been defined in 1958 and generally accepted as a drug complication since the mid-1960s, many clinicians have not been acutely aware of the high prevalence of tardive dyskinesia in patients receiving antipsychotic drugs over long periods. Recent hospital studies suggest that 35 to 55 percent of patients on long-term antipsychotic medications manifest evidence of tardive dyskinesia, and surveys of outpatient medication clinics find at least suggestive evidence of tardive dyskinesia in 30 to 45 percent of patients. Many cases have been described following short-term drug use, but the incidence is high only after a year or longer on antipsychotic medication. Since the risk of tardive dyskinesia increases with age and duration of treatment, risk/benefit ratios have to be recalculated over time.

The cause of tardive dyskinesia is by no means established, although it is clear that neuroleptic drugs play a key role. These drugs induce dopaminergic supersensitivity in animals and apparently in man, epidemiological evidence implicates the drugs in tardive dyskinesia, and drug/involuntary movement interactions further establish a causative role. However, a few patients develop dyskinesia after brief treatment, and many patients do not develop the disorder despite years and years of neuroleptics.

Understanding the cause of tardive dyskinesia is complicated further by the fact that age increases vulnerability to movement disorders generally, including tardive dyskinesia. Also, abnormal movements have been reported in schizophrenia well before the drug treatment era, and the differential diagnosis between low prevalent schizophrenic abnormal movements and high prevalent tardive dyskinesia is not always easy to establish. Nevertheless, a working hypothesis postulates an imbalance between cholinergic (↑) and dopaminergic (↓) function in tardive dyskinesia, and experimental therapeutics aimed at increasing cholinergic activity with choline or lecithin have produced encouraging results.[27,28] Because of the many variables influencing the onset of dyskinesia, however, it is assumed that a number of factors are involved in its etiology.

Some forms of tardive dyskinesia are reversible following drug discontinuation; therefore, it is especially important for the clinician to observe the face, mouth, tongue, and extremities of patients frequently and carefully in order to detect early signs. Drug discontinuation for a period of about four weeks can reveal covert dyskinesias where abnormal movements are being suppressed by dopamine-blocking neuroleptic drugs. The feasibility and usefulness of this procedure in outpatients has been demonstrated.[29]

In any patient with early signs of tardive dyskinesia, every effort should be made to reverse the syndrome with drug reduction and discontinuation. The movement disorder may worsen acutely, but the suppression of symptoms with ever increasing dosages buys a short-term gain at a long-term cost. We do not yet know how many early cases will reverse spontaneously on drug discontinuation or reduction. It is clear, however, that most (not all) patients with chronic tardive dyskinesia will probably have irreversible syndromes, and every effort is required to reduce the prevalence by more judicious use of medication, particularly employing minimal effective dosage level, curtailing the duration of treatment, and not continuing chronic, nonresponsive patients willy–nilly on medication.[30] Although the clinical need for such caution is the most important consideration, litigation and administrative fiat will further emphasize caution in the use of antipsychotic drugs, and there is a danger of backlash which will unduly restrict pharmacotherapeutics.

Informed consent is an ethic governing all clinical interventions, and it is a mistake to think that only somatic treatments come under informed consent considerations. However, concerning antipsychotic drugs, some particular issues should be emphasized. The benefit–risk ratio in short-term treatment with these drugs is so advantageous that oral informed consent seems sufficient. However, benefits and risks change with duration of treatment, and written informed consent in patients remaining on medication for longer than six to twelve months may be useful to all concerned. Such informed consent would especially note the risk of tardive dyskinesia with medication and the risk of psychotic exacerbation without it.

7. Polypharmacy has justifiably received a bad name because it ordinarily denotes ill-informed mixing of medication. However, the clinician will often find patients with whom it seems wise to use multiple drugs for specific purposes. For example, in a schizophrenic patient who cannot sleep and is sensitive to the extrapyramidal side effects of antipsychotics, the clinician may wish to use a drug with sedative side effects and a low profile of extrapyramidal side effects as evening medication, while using smaller doses of nonsedating neuroleptics during the day. A schizophrenic patient with severe depression may be a good candidate for antidepressant medication. The clinician may wish to use prophylactic antipsychotic medication concomitantly to reduce risk of a drug-induced psychotic exacerbation. The clinician using depot decanoate preparations for maintenance may also wish to use oral preparations for targeted use. Careful thought and adequate recorded documentation of the reasons for multiple drug treatment are needed to ensure its justification, to avoid criticism, and to inform the patient's future clinicians of the rationale involved.

8. The clinician must identify schizophrenic patients who might profit from pharmacotherapy other than antipsychotic medication. Severe depression in schizophrenic patients and psychotic depression confused with schizophrenia have pharmacological requirements which differ from those of schizophrenia itself. Similarly, patients with manic features to their schizophrenia, or manic patients mistakenly considered schizophrenic, may benefit from lithium maintenance.

The problem in assuming specific drug treatment–diagnosis links is further complicated by the fact that we do not yet have a satisfactory nosology for the functional psychoses, and acute psychotic illnesses are given many names including acute schizophrenic reaction, reactive psychoses, schizoaffective psychoses, episodic psychoses, and cycloid psychoses. Some such patients are lithium-responsive; others appear to have an episodic dyscontrol syndrome conceptualized as limbic ictus and are responsive to antiseizure medication.[31]

For these reasons, the doctor is encouraged to be adventurous in seeking the best drug(s) for each patient. Psychopharmacology has not yet produced a drug the therapeutic effect of which is specific to one class of illness. A patient who meets criteria for a diagnosis of schizophrenia but has some manic features and a family history of affective disorder certainly deserves a trial on lithium. A good response may or may not challenge the original diagnosis, but in either case we may have achieved better therapy at less risk. And, of course, the clinician must also keep in mind the fact that a therapeutic response to antipsychotic medication does not confirm a diagnosis of schizophrenia!

9. New developments in neuropsychopharmacology are promising, and the clinician can reasonably anticipate development of nonneuroleptic antipsychotic medication (see Chapter 7).

NONPHARMACOLOGICAL SOMATIC TREATMENTS

The aims of this book preclude any extensive consideration of all potential treatment modalities for schizophrenia, whether psychosocial or somatic in nature. Hence, we will only comment briefly on somatic treatments other than medication. Currently, the most important somatic modality besides medication is electroconvulsive therapy. There have always been outspoken advocates of ECT for schizophrenia, but there are very few controlled studies of its use in this disorder. One such study does lend some support to the efficacy of this treatment.[32] Clinicians using ECT often claim that it is most effective in acute cases, but acute onset, good prognosis cases show a more favorable course of illness than process and chronic schizophrenia, no matter what treatments are or are not given.

It is unfortunate that hard data cannot shape opinions concerning ECT, but little information is available. Given this situation, we think it prudent to limit ECT in treating schizophrenia for several reasons. First, there is no evidence that it is curative in any sense beyond the type of symptom remission associated with antipsychotic drugs. Second, it is psychologically complicated to apply a procedure shrouded with mystery and punitiveness in psychotic and often resistant patients. Third, if bilateral ECT is used, one would predict that confusion and memory impediments might have a deleterious effect on an important area of function not compromised by the disorder (the clear sensorium!).

Even in affective disorders with which more impressive evidence of efficacy is available, planning the therapeutic use of ECT is influenced by professional attitude, patient fears, public policy, litigation, etc. For schizophrenic patients, our personal view is to limit ECT treatment to affective disturbance components of illness clearly demonstrated as resistant to pharmacological and psychotherapeutic intervention in the particular patient and to acute management of excited or catatonic behavior in very rare circumstances.

Psychosurgery for schizophrenia is a past tragedy and is presently used in only a few centers. One cannot exclude the possibility of a benefit worth the risk with discrete surgery for some patients, but guidelines are not adequate for defining the patient population or the surgical procedure at this date. It is arguable whether schizophrenic subjects should even be considered for such treatment in carefully supervised and designed clinical investigations, and we certainly object to other clinical application of psychosurgery for schizophrenic patients.

Hemodialysis and orthomolecular treatments are currently the focus of considerable attention and curiosity. The orthomolecular approaches have had years in which to establish a scientific basis for clinical application and have been found wanting. Our view of the extensive data is that the various orthomolecular approaches are without proven effectiveness. Whether some minor subtypes of schizophrenia will prove to receive therapeutic benefit from orthomolecular treatment cannot be settled with present evidence.[33]

Hemodialysis, on the other hand, has only recently begun to develop a base of clinical studies from which to make a judgment regarding therapeutic efficacy. The claims for symptomatic and social cures by Wagemaker and Cade[34] seem implausible to the clinician deeply invested in a complex interactive developmental model of the illness and mindful of the multitude of dysfunctional areas in the chronic schizophrenic patient. Although the artificial kidneys can remove some substances not excreted by the functioning human kidney, it is not immediately obvious why hemodialysis should be beneficial to the schizophrenic patient with good renal function. Furthermore, there are numerous reports of psychotic experiences arising in the course of hemodialysis and other reports of schizophrenic patients who undergo dialysis (because of renal pathology) and fail to improve psychiatrically. Conclusions concerning the therapeutic efficacy of hemodialysis must await the results of controlled studies, and implementation as a nonexperimental treatment is not now justified.

GENERAL CONSIDERATIONS REGARDING NEW TREATMENTS

Any clinician's receptivity to a new treatment approach will be partially determined by the model of illness to which he or she subscribes, personal attitudes towards the patient, and the theoretical nature of etiological assumptions. It often goes unnoticed that simple factors play a major role in treatment proclivities. For example, a doctor personally offended by abusive language and lack of respect may be more receptive to somatic innovations than talking therapies. Another comparably trained clinician who enjoys ambiguity and symbolic language may embrace psychotherapeutic innovations and be disinclined towards somatic treatments. Also, the professional who emphasizes genetic etiology is likely to be especially interested in biochemical modalities, while those who focus on family environment will be intuitively in tune with psychological interventions. Such dichotomies, although founded on bias, do have some impact on the acceptance of new treatments.

Taking these personal and professional factors into account, can we establish general guidelines useful to clinicians in deciding when and what therapeutic innovation to apply in practice? Or, to put it more pungently, what should the doctor do until the data come? Two rules of thumb are applicable for clinical implementation of new or unproven treatments. First, we believe new treatments that are not intuitively understandable and may involve significant hazard or expense should be avoided until they are proved safe and effective. These considerations have nothing to do with potential efficacy, but it is wise for the clinician to await proof of therapeutic benefit and safety before applying these treatments clinically. Hemodialysis is illustrative, for it is not intuitively obvious why an artificial kidney should cure schizophrenia in patients with normal kidneys. The risks of treatment are considerable, and the circumstances and expense are extraordinary. The nonintuitive, potentially hazardous category of treatment should be taken seriously by the theoretician and clinical investigator, but the practicing clinician requires the results of their studies to determine what, if any, applicability such new treatments have to those people for whom he has accepted clinical responsibility.

The second rule of thumb involves intuitively based treatments which can occur in nonextraordinary circumstances with minimal risk. Many of the psychosocial treatment approaches fall into this category. We have complained about the unfortunate lack of good data concerning therapeutic efficacy of interpersonal strategies, but we accept their application by the clinician at present because of the intuitive rationale and the body of clinical observation supportive of these treatments. For example, occupational counseling is sensible in a population where two-thirds of the discharged patients are unemployed. When careful studies are conducted, they may prove that occupational counseling and vocational rehabilitation have a negligible effect on work functioning and hence might be abandoned. But it seems wise to incorporate such commonsense endeavors as social skills training, approaching problems in interpersonal relationships with psychotherapy, or enhancing work functioning with occupational counseling in our therapeutic armamentarium, until such time as there is good evidence that they have no effect. The risks seem minimal unless such means are used to the exclusion of other treatments or are applied without good clinical sense.

We realize that this dichotomy is strained and that not all psychosocial treatments are intuitive, safe, or inexpensive. A therapeutic relationship for socially isolated and perplexed patients will seem sensible to most clinicians, but psychoanalytic exploration of intrapsychic conflict will be intuitively appealing only to those who believe psychological conflict relevant to schizophrenia. Nevertheless, we believe the clinician has a responsibility for using common sense to employ a wide range of potentially therapeutic endeavors on behalf of the schizophrenic patient but that those treatments which do not have an intuitive rationale or may be dangerous should be avoided until a firm body of evidence supporting them is established. Concern about depriving patients of such treatments when they have proven effective will be minimized if it is appreciated that somatic interventions lend themselves to crisp scientific evaluation and those found therapeutically efficacious will find their way to the clinical market place.

SUMMARY

The treatment of schizophrenic patients should be based on an appreciation of the complexity of this uniquely human disorder, a realization that no disease specific or comprehensive therapeutic modality exists for schizophrenia, and the recognition that diagnosis and subtype designations are only first steps in organizing treatment-relevant data. Intelligent treatment planning eventually rests on a detailed and individualized understanding of the patient's experiences, past history, strengths and weaknesses, psychosocial context of illness, prognosis, and response to previous therapeutic initiatives.

We have been alarmed by today's nearly exclusive emphasis on rapid symptom remission. Enlightened treatment of the schizophrenic patient requires the clinician to use techniques and knowledge from diverse sources. Therapeutic goals must extend far beyond achievement of symptom relief and prevention of relapse and rehospitalization. The most devastating aspect of much schizophrenia is the defect state with its incapacities in social, work, and psychological function. Unidimensional therapeutics are too narrow for schizophrenia and cause clinicians and investigators to underemphasize major areas of dysfunction which fall outside the small range of therapeutic effects of any single treatment.

RECOMMENDED READING

Davis, J., Schaffer, C., Killian, G., Kinard, C., and Chan, C. Important issues in the drug treatment of schizophrenia. *Schizophrenia Bulletin*, 1980, 6:70–87.
May, P. Schizophrenia: Evaluation of treatment. In: *Comprehensive Textbook of Psychiatry*, Vol. 2, Freedman, A., Kaplan, H., and Sadock, B. (eds.). Baltimore: Williams and Wilkins, 1975, 955–982.
Mosher, L., and Gunderson, J. Group, family, milieu, and community support systems treatment for schizophrenia. In: *Disorders of the schizophrenic syndrome*, Bellak, L. New York: Basic Books, 1979, 399–452.
Scott, R. D., and Ashworth, P. The shadow of the ancestor. *British Journal of Medical Psychology*, 1969, 42:13–32.

REFERENCES

1. Barton, R. *Institutional neurosis*. Bristol: Wright, 1959.
2. Wing, J., and Brown, G. *Institutionalism and schizophrenia*. Cambridge: Cambridge University Press, 1970.
3. Hogarty, G., Goldberg, S., Schooler, N., Ulrich, R. *et al.* Drugs and sociotherapy in the aftercare of schizophrenic patients. *Archives of General Psychiatry*, 1974, 131:603–608.
4. Clausen, J. The impact of mental illness: A 20-year follow-up. In: *Life history*

research in psychopathology, Vol. 4, Wirt, R. D., Winokur, G., and Roff, M. (eds.). Minneapolis: University of Minnesota Press, 1976, 270–289.

5. Lamb, H., and Goertzel, V. Discharged mental patients—are they really in the community? *Archives of General Psychiatry*, 1971, 24:29–34.

6. Glick, I., Hargreaves, W., Raskin, M., et al. Short versus long hospitalization. II. Results for schizophrenic inpatients. *American Journal of Psychiatry*, 1975, 132:385–390.

7. Phipps, L. The impact of psychiatric hospitalization on the spouse of the identified patient. Unpublished master's thesis, School of Nursing, University of Rochester, Rochester, NY, 1976.

8. Mosher, L., and Keith, S. Research on the psychosocial treatment of schizophrenia: A summary report. *American Journal of Psychiatry*, 1979, 136:623–631.

9. Strauss, J. S., Kokes, R. F., Ritzler, B. A., Harder, D. W., and VanOrd, A. Patterns of disorder in first admission psychiatric patients. *Journal of Nervous and Mental Disease*, 1978, 166(9):611–625.

10. Heinrichs, D.W., and Carpenter, W. T., Jr. The efficacy of individual psychotherapy: A perspective and review emphasizing controlled outcome studies. In: *The American Handbook of Psychiatry*, Vol. 7, Arieti, S., and Brodie, H. K. (eds.). New York: Basic Books in press.

11. McGlashan, T. H., and Carpenter, W. T., Jr. Affective symptoms and the diagnosis of schizophrenia. *Schizophrenia Bulletin*, 1979, 5(4):547–553.

12. Carpenter, W. T., Jr., and Heinrichs, D. The role for psychodynamic psychiatry in the treatment of schizophrenic patients. In: *Psychotherapy of Schizophrenia*, Strauss, J. S., Bowers, M., Downey, T. W. *et al.* (eds.). New York: Plenum, 1980.

13. Bleuler, M. *The schizophrenic disorders: Long-term patient and family studies.* Translated by S. M. Clemens. New Haven: Yale University Press, 1978.

14. Ciompi, L. The natural history of schizophrenia in the long term. *British Journal of Psychiatry*, 1980, 136:413–420.

15. Strauss, J. S., Loevsky, L., Glazer, W., and Leaf, P. Organizing the complexities of schizophrenia. *Journal of Nervous and Mental Disease*, in press.

16. O'Brien, C. Group therapy for schizophrenia. *Schizophrenia Bulletin*, 1975, 13:119–130.

17. Vaughn, C., and Leff, J. The influence of family and social factors on the course of psychiatric illness. *British Journal of Psychiatry*, 1976, 139:125–137.

18. Mosher, L., and Gunderson, G. Group, family, milieu and community support systems treatment for schizophrenia. In: *Disorders of the schizophrenic syndrome*, Bellak, L. New York: Basic Books, 1979, 399–452.

19. Goldstein, M. J., Rodnick, E. H., Evans, J. R., May, R. A., and Steinberg, M. R. Drug and family therapy in the aftercare of acute schizophrenics. *Archives of General Psychiatry*, 1978, 35:1169–1177.

20. Paul G. Comprehensive psychosocial treatment: Beyond traditional psychotherapy. In: *The psychotherapy of schizophrenia*, Strauss, J. S., Bowers, M., Downey, T. W. *et al.* (eds.). New York: Plenum, 1980.

21. Liberman, R. P., Wallace, C. J., Vaughn, C. E. *et al.* Social and family factors in the course of schizophrenia: Toward an interpersonal problem-solving

therapy for schizophrenics and their families. In: *The psychotherapy of schizophrenia*, Strauss, J. S., Bowers, M., Downey, T. W. *et al.* (eds.). New York: Plenum, 1980.

22. Davis, J., Schaffer, C., Killian, G., Kinard, C., and Chan, C. Important issues in the drug treatment of schizophrenia. *Schizophrenia Bulletin*, 1980, 6:70–87.

23. Hogarty, G. E., Goldberg, S., and Schooler, N. Drugs and sociotherapy in the aftercare of schizophrenia: A review. In: *Drugs in combination with other therapies*, Greenblatt, M. (ed.). New York: Grune & Stratton, 1975.

24. Crane, G. E. Risks of long-term therapy with neuroleptic drugs. In: *Antipsychotic drugs: Pharmacodynamics and pharmacokinetics, Wenner-Gren International Symposium Series*, Vol. 25, Unvas, B., and Zotterman, Y. (eds.). Elmsford, NY: Pergamon Press, 1976.

25. Gardos, G., and Cole, J. O. Overview: Public health issues in tardive dyskinesia. *American Journal of Psychiatry*, 1980, 137:776–781.

26. Carpenter, W. T., Jr., and Rudo, A. Tardive dyskinesia: A major risk of neuroleptic drugs. *Behavioral Medicine*, July, 1979, 33–37.

27. Davis, K., Berger, P., and Hollister, L. Choline for tardive dyskinesia. *The New England Journal of Medicine*, 1975, 293:152.

28. Gelenberg, A. J., Doller-Wojcik, J. E., and Growdon, J. H. Choline and lecithin in the treatment of tardive dyskinesia: Preliminary results from a pilot study. *American Journal of Psychiatry*, 1979, 136:772–776.

29. Carpenter, W. T., Jr., Rey, A. C., and Stephens, J. H. Covert dyskinesia in ambulatory schizophrenia. *The Lancet*, July 26, 1980, 8187:212–213.

30. Gardos, G., and Cole, J. O. Maintenance antipsychotic therapy: Is the cure worse than the disease? *American Journal of Psychiatry*, 1976, 133:32–36.

31. Monroe, R. R. *Episodic behavioral disorders*. Cambridge: Harvard University Press, 1970.

32. May, P., and Tuma, H. Follow-up study of the results of treatment of schizophrenia. In: *Evaluation of psychological therapies*, Spitzer, R., and Klein, D. (eds.). Baltimore: Johns Hopkins University Press, 1976, 256–284.

33. Ban, T. A., and Lehmann, H. E. Nicotinic acid in the treatment of schizophrenia, Part 2. *Canadian Psychiatric Association Journal*, 1976, 20:103–112.

34. Wagemaker, H., and Cade, R. The use of hemodialysis in chronic schizophrenia. *American Journal of Psychiatry*, 1977, 134:684–685.

The Clinical–Legal Interface in Schizophrenia

Administrative, legislative, and judicial considerations are increasingly affecting clinical care and research. Policies, laws, and judgments (and even the threat of future actions) now influence treatment and investigations involving schizophrenic patients. This review is not comprehensive, nor are the conclusions necessarily legally elegant. Rather, we express a point of view on several issues of concern to the clinician and investigator, issues in which the clinician's vantage as care-giving expert and patient advocate is underrepresented in public deliberations attempting to provide safeguards against very real problems.

INFORMED CONSENT

Clinicians engaged in the diagnosis and treatment of patients and in human experimental work are obliged to follow the ethical principles that fall under the rubric of informed consent. Three such principles are particularly crucial: that the patient have the necessary basic information regarding a treatment or procedure and its alternatives; that he/she understand the risk and benefit implications of the treatment or procedure; and that there be an absence of coercion.

It is by default that the public and many professionals believe that informed consent is a set of special considerations relevant only to research with human subjects and to a few noteworthy treatment procedures such as surgery and ECT. In fact, the ordinary provision of treatment requires the clinician to inform the patient of anticipated benefits and possible risks and provide him or her with a reasonable view of alternative approaches. This need not be a legalistic procedure requiring written documentation in most instances; some even argue that the more formal aspects of informed consent are for the protection of institutions and clinicians rather than for patients.[1]

Recent developments in clinical practice relevant to the care of schizophrenic patients will cause the prudent clinician to follow the principles of informed consent even for ordinary treatment procedures. The risk of neurological complications associated with long-term use of neuroleptic drugs, for example, presents visible risk associated with a treatment of demonstrated efficacy. The risk is greater in the elderly, in those patients with CNS impairment, and in patients who have received prolonged neuroleptic treatment. For this modality, the risk–benefit ratio is quite different in the acute stage, as opposed to later stages of treatment. In the early stages, expectation of benefit is high and risk low. However, when treatment is prolonged, both benefit and risk considerations alter remarkably, and informed consent processes must be reinitiated.

This example reflects a common mistake made with many treatments: that the clinician conceptualizes a simple continuation of an already established modality without noting the shift in the risk–benefit profile. Alternative approaches with neuroleptics include the more judicious and targeted use of medication or prolonged periods of treatment without medication. There are also risks and benefits associated with these approaches, and the clinician must be careful to specify these issues in discussing such alternatives. It is rarely that we can provide risk-free clinical care, and no treatment alternatives carry the least acceptable benefit/risk ratios!

Informed consent relevant to various psychosocial treatments receives particularly scant attention. Psychosocial therapeutic approaches have alternatives with which the patient should be familiar, and it is not justifiable to assume that the risks are inconsequential. Furthermore, some clinicians with a particular therapeutic philosophy present treatments as though they were mutually exclusive. While the field awaits more precise information on the optimal integration of various treatment modalities, it is usually unwarranted to advise patients that a single therapeutic approach must be selected to the exclusion of others.

Of more general concern is the disconcerting body of opinion which holds that patients with psychotic experiences are not competent to participate in informed consent processes. "How," it is asked, "can a patient who believes he is being poisoned by medication become an informed and reasonable advocate on his own behalf?" This position has led to proposed special protection for schizophrenic patients which subject them to protections under the law similar to those established for the mentally retarded, prisoners, and children. We believe this position is invalid and hold that efforts suggested to resolve this problem[2] should be supported and that informed consent should be and can be pursued with schizophrenic patients.

Our view is based on two premises. The first is a realistic rather than idealized appraisal of the quality of informed consent in other patient populations and other medical circumstances. Many problems intrinsic in the doctor–patient relationship at times interfere with successful informing of the patient and self-advocacy by the patient.[3] Impediments include high esteem in which the doctor may be held, the urgency with which the patient seeks care, the expectation that the doctor will act in the patient's best interest, the willingness to yield to a socially sanctioned expert's opinion, and external (e.g., family) pressures to follow the doctor's orders. Informed consent is difficult in all medical settings, and special considerations are relevant to many patient populations. The severely depressed patient may secretly wish to die and be willing to accept any procedure offered on entirely irrational grounds. A lower socioeconomic class surgical patient may have been reared with such rigid respect for authority that he dare not challenge the medical expert, and an upper-middle-class housewife may be so enamored of her physician as to preclude self-advocacy.

Given these problems, the second part of the argument calls attention to the capacity of psychotic patients to maintain some aspects of reality testing, receptivity to information, and self-protection. The patient's mental status often fluctuates considerably, and the clinician skilled at engaging psychotic patients in the interpersonal context of a therapeutic relationship will find many moments of rational thinking and behavior. Besides this consideration, informed consent must be conceptualized as a process that takes place at multiple points in time and that need not rely exclusively on the doctor/patient dyad. Hence, group discussions, family discussions, and discussion with nurses and with other patients will gradually increase the patient's store of information concerning risks and benefits of various treatment approaches and enable the patient to participate more effectively in the informed consent process.[4]

Finally, treatment for schizophrenic patients often lasts for an extended time, and there are many periods during which the patient is free or relatively free of psychotic distortions during which an exchange of information and self-advocacy can take place. While perhaps not legally significant, retrospective consideration of treatment decisions is personally meaningful, and prospective consideration of treatment alternatives for future psychotic episodes can be undertaken.

PROTECTION OF SUBJECTS IN INVESTIGATIVE WORK

Protection of subjects involves procedures and considerations beyond informed consent. Since these rarely impact directly on the practitioner, clinicians and patients are often unaware of the deleterious effects of well-intentioned regulations. Clinical investigators are now faced with a multitude of laws, administrative policies, and judicial actions which attempt to specify the circumstances of investigative work. While all parties believe proper protection of subjects requires regulation and review, it is not so readily appreciated that the maze of overlapping requirements, penalties and participants is costly and discourages the acquisition of new knowledge so vital to patient welfare. The public debate of these issues is often one-sided, lacking adequate input from informed patients, health advocacy groups, and clinicians. Hence, debate centers extensively around preventing abuse without simultaneously protecting the process of gaining new information. For example, new laws or regulations intended to effect a certain protection may be enacted without anyone's realizing that protections are already in place and that wanton abuse is already minimized. Proposals, for example, to provide consent auditors who would constitute a cumbersome and expensive bureaucracy supervising the doctor–patient relationship may impose adversarial relationships which undermine investigative work without actually significantly increasing the protection of subjects. This is paralleled in some clinical settings in which ordinary matters of treatment such as hospital status and the administration of medication are routinely exposed to adversarial rather than caretaking considerations.

The clinician can provide badly needed input in the public discussions of protection for human subjects. In the first place, professional ethics and the American Constitution place preeminent emphasis on the patient's rights. The physician and clinical investigator are ethically guided, morally required, and institutionally reviewed concerning their respect for, and advocacy of, patient well-being. In general, clinicians and clinical investigators remain the professionals best trained to be advocates on the patient's behalf. The clinician should resist the tendency of some segments of the public to view the relationship as primarily adversarial or the doctor's role as being largely undermined by conflict of interest.

In the second place, it should be appreciated that conflicting rights exist wherever protection of the individual subject is concerned. If there is a right to treatment, then it follows that those charged with the responsibility of providing treatment are entitled to knowledge of effective therapeutics. The consequent necessity for treatment research need not ever override the individual's right to decline participation in research, but procedures which overprotect the individual to the clear detriment of investigative efforts are not balancing the various needs implied in the right to treatment. Schizophrenic patients, particularly, are entitled to greater knowledge regarding the cause, diagnosis, and treatment of their disorders, and unwarranted impediments to the acquisition of new knowledge further deprive this already socially and individually disadvantaged group. One of the pleasures of clinical research that might surprise many cynics is to find how common it is for patients and their families to want altruistically to participate, in order to help others avoid the kinds of problems from which they themselves have suffered.

The individual's right to be adequately informed and protected regarding participation in investigative work is the primary consideration governing the ethics of clinical research. The clinician and clinical investigator have crucial roles in assuring the patient's capacity for choice and self-protection. This role should not be abrogated. Investigators' proposals are and should be scrutinized by colleagues and review groups, and the nature of informed consent should be specified and the patient's privilege of nonparticipation protected. But the clinician should not fail to press on the public's attention the desperate need for information relevant to etiology, diagnosis, and treatment of schizophrenia, nor should patients or citizen advocates fail to press for clinical research and against the domination of ignorance.

RIGHT TO TREATMENT

Although professional considerations traditionally suggest that patients are entitled to treatment, some judicial opinions have recently brought this issue under formal scrutiny. It is clear that many factors in various societies combine to limit treatment opportunities, and at times health leaders have been unduly tolerant of shortcomings. The housing of chronic schizophrenic patients in crowded, understaffed custodial environments is a glaring example. Comments here are restricted to several instances in which legal and clinical perspectives are discordant.

The legal implications of voluntary and involuntary status are now directly affecting clinical care decisions and the potential for providing treatment. From a professional perspective, patients are entitled to good clinical care regardless of their legal status, and our responsibility is not lessened by voluntary status.

It is also intellectually indefensible to define treatment of schizophrenia so narrowly that some clinicians responsible for care of involuntarily admitted patients, and some administrators responsible for the hospitals in which such care is provided, fear that they will be vulnerable to charges of withholding treatment unless medication is used. The comments in earlier sections of this book should make it clear that treatment must be conceptualized broadly, that an individual's needs vary from time to time, and that multiple modalities are available. The clinician, of course, should resist whatever pressures may coerce him to apply any treatment unwisely. Of more profound consequence, however, is the need for psychiatric practitioners to inform administrators, the judiciary, and any third parties who may be financially responsible for the patient of the range of therapeutic modalities applicable in patients diagnosed as schizophrenic.

Other popularized issues regarding treatment decisions, such as the use of the least restrictive environment, forcible administration of medication, and prohibition of the use of ECT, have led to policies and judgments which often fail to reflect clinical acumen and scientific fact. The focus on the least restrictive environment rather than on the most therapeutic environment, for example, reflects the imprimatur of the judiciary and body politic, more than psychiatric judgment. Abuses, neglect, and negligence occur and nonmedical remedies must be available, but we are concerned with the inadequate representation of clinical considerations in these decisions.

Many clinicians are hesitant to assume the role of expert witness in judicial proceedings, feeling (among other things) inexperienced and unprepared to enter debate on adversarial territory. However, the forensically naive clinical expert may be especially persuasive in portraying clinical care issues from the vantage of health needs rather than that of the legal framework. A lawyer once explained that as forensically experienced psychiatrists begin thinking and talking in the language of the court, the judges are less likely to be influenced, because they already are familiar with those arguments. However, they may be deeply impressed by a clinician's testimony which compels the judiciary to think in terms that reflect clinical contingencies. In this regard, it is critical for the practicing clinician to remember that he cannot delegate his responsibilities to a court of law and that only the clinician can diagnose and treat. A simple case in point is the responsibility for defining when a clinical emergency exists (hence permitting certain curtailments of freedom). Clinicians are responsible for determining the presence of an emergency, although from time to time a court may review how the clinician reached this judgment and what actions he took based on this judgment.

The discomfort of many clinicians faced with public inquiries may be partially explained by a feeling that they must adopt the rules and language of another system. In many instances, the clinician's strength lies in maintaining the concepts, guidelines, and language of his field. The adversarial pursuit of "facts" is not always suited to understanding the ambiguities and uncertainties of clinical processes.

VIOLENCE IN SCHIZOPHRENIA AND ITS LEGAL IMPLICATIONS

When schizophrenic persons act in an antisocial way, the important legal issue of responsibility is raised. In order to consider this issue, it is crucial first to note whether such behavior is in fact intrinsic to this disorder. Many assume that the schizophrenic individual is prone to crimes of violence, but available epidemiological data are conflicting.[5-7] The most common interpretations of these data are (a) schizophrenic patients are no more likely to commit crimes of violence than the general population; and (b) schizophrenic patients may be involved in violence slightly in excess of population norms.

Although homicide is, of course, the most feared, real or threatened violence at less drastic levels is sometimes associated with psychosis and tends particularly to affect the family and caretakers intimately involved with some schizophrenic patients. While no prevalence figures are available, belligerence, impulsivity, and physical altercations are sufficiently common to create a high degree of tension in some households, residential treatment settings, and hospitals. Although serious harm is infrequent, it causes an understandable apprehension in some patients and in settings routinely responsible for management and treatment of psychotic patients.

Despite these important concerns, available data do not begin to justify society's undue fear of schizophrenic patients. Public concern for criminal violence in schizophrenia is high and directly impedes implementation of some aspects of long-term treatment (e.g., reduced employment opportunities, zoning laws preventing shared residential quarters for patients). The apprehension of violence from schizophrenic patients is heightened by instances of bizarre and psychotic homicidal behavior by popular images (e.g., "homicidal maniac"), movies (e.g., *Psycho*), and the frequent use of the insanity plea, all reinforcing the myth of schizophrenia as a public hazard. It appears to be human nature to fear that which is unknown, and stereotyping of disenfranchised groups is usually harsh and forbidding. This process influences attitudes toward schizophrenic patients well beyond a reasonable degree.

These data and social beliefs have major implications for the use of insanity as a defense in murder trials. There are unequivocal instances in which severe, violent, and destructive behavior is explicable in terms of psychotic ideation, irresistible impulsivity, and an inability to appreciate ordinary social restraints. In such instances, the application of the medical model rather than a social or legal model for understanding the disordered behavior and for guiding society's response to the deviant individual appears the most valid. However, the widespread use of the insanity plea extends medical explanations for antisocial behavior far beyond the explanatory power of a scientifically validated medical model. Excessive use of this plea may eventually eliminate its availability to those schizophrenic individuals whose violence is explicable in terms of psychotic experience. Such a person needs the insanity defense to provide the most therapeutic and benevolent response of society compatible with providing public security. In this regard it can also be noted that schizophrenic patients do many things not explicable in terms of their illness, including acts of violence. A valid diagnosis of schizophrenia does not automatically provide a valid explanation for all deviant behavior observed in the individual.

SUMMARY

The clinical–legal interface in schizophrenia affects many aspects of treatment and research. Informed consent, the right to treatment, the use of restraint in treatment environments, and concern for violence are all important. These considerations are influenced by stereotypes and over-simplification. Even during psychosis, aspects of rational functioning may persist. From the clinical vantage, conflicting "rights" can often be perceived. Patients are entitled to optimal treatment as well as to the least restrictive environment, to new knowledge (derived of necessity from research) of their illness as well as to protection from poor treatment and exploitation. A balance has not been achieved in the public debate of these issues, and clinicians have failed to advocate their models vigorously in nonclinical forums.

RECOMMENDED READING

Halleck, S. L. *Law in the practice of psychiatry: A handbook for clinicians.* New York: Plenum, 1980.

Romano, J. Reflections on informed consent. *Archives of General Psychiatry,* 1974, 30:129–135.

Stone, A. A. Informed consent: Special problems for psychiatry. *Hospital and Community Psychiatry,* 1979, 30(5):321–327.

REFERENCES

1. Loftus, E. F., and Fries, J. F. Informed consent may be hazardous to health. *Science,* 1979, 204:4388.
2. Roth, L. H., Meisel, A., and Lidz, C. Tests of competency to consent to treatment. *American Journal of Psychiatry,* 1977, 134:279–284.
3. Carpenter, W. T., Jr. A new setting for informed consent. *The Lancet,* 1974, 1:500–501.
4. Carpenter, W. T., Jr., and Langsner, C. A. The nurse's role in informed consent. *Nursing Times,* 1975, 71:1049–1051.
5. Sosowsky, L. Crime and violence among mental patients reconsidered in view of new legal relationship between state and mentally ill. *American Journal of Psychiatry,* 1978, 135:33–42.
6. Report of the Task Panel on Legal and Ethical Issues: President's Commission on Mental Health, Vol. 4. Washington, D.C.: U.S. Government Printing Office, 1978.
7. Gulevich, G., and Bourne, P. Mental illness and violence. In: *Violence and the struggle for existence,* Daniels, D., Gulula, M., and Ochberg, F. Boston: Little, Brown, 1970.

CHAPTER 12

In Conclusion

PRINCIPLES UNDERLYING TREATMENT, RESEARCH, AND UNDERSTANDING OF SCHIZOPHRENIA

In the preceding chapters, we have described a model for synthesizing information relevant to the concept of schizophrenia and useful to the clinician responsible for the care and study of patients. We have emphasized the importance of a phenomenological, rather than a narrow descriptive, basis for diagnosis and treatment and the necessity of a combined biological, psychological, and social foundation for considering etiology, pathogenesis, and treatment. In closing, we will state a few salient principles and admonitions that we believe to be crucial for the investigation, understanding, and clinical care of schizophrenic patients.

INDIVIDUALS, NOT COHORTS, HAVE SCHIZOPHRENIA

Psychiatrists and other mental health professionals are prepared by training and clinical tasks to remain sensitive to the individuality of each patient and to conceptualize illness within the context of the patient's attributes, circumstances, and environment. Personal and environmental factors have a profound influence on the form, substance, and eventual consequences of illness. Nonetheless, the principle of individuality is often violated, and patients are diagnosed and treated in the absence of sufficient personal data. Treatment programs often ignore the patient's strengths and fail to relate to the broad range of human functioning potentially compromised by schizophrenic illness and society's reaction to that illness.

Heterogeneity of patients classified as schizophrenic is almost the hallmark of the disorder; yet, the modal schizophrenic patient is often processed through the health care system with surprisingly little attention paid to him or her as an individual and with unwarranted assumptions that the individual represents primarily one case in a homogeneous group phenomenon. To know that a patient fits in a diagnostic niche is not sufficient information on which to base clinical care decisions, and treatment and diagnosis of the schizophrenic patient will be severely compromised in any circumstance in which the patient's individuality is ignored.

THE CLINICIAN/PATIENT RELATIONSHIP IS INDISPENSIBLE TO CLINICAL CARE

Our primary method for gaining information about another person's experiences is in the context of an informative relationship which fosters the transfer of information on both a cognitive and empathic level. We have emphasized the importance of a solid phenomenological basis for diagnostic and treatment decisions. To focus only on a few conspicuous features of illness and remain uninformed concerning the breadth and depth of the psychopathology, strengths, and environmental conditions is to make a mockery of classification and to base treatment, research, and concepts on a narrow and distorted base.

The clinical/therapeutic relationship is an ongoing process which continually generates new information and reconsideration of diagnostic and treatment decisions. This process also provides a reasonable opportunity for the patient to understand and collaborate in treatment and fosters an ongoing assessment of therapeutic effects. The clinical/ therapeutic relationship enables early recognition of decompensation, identification of areas of vulnerability, and circumstances of particular stress. The interpersonal aspect of the clinical relationship is as important to somatic treatment as it is to psychosocial treatment, and we advocate this as a principle in clinical care regardless of the therapeutic philosophy espoused by the treating clinician.

However, the health care networks available to the average schizophrenic patient (unemployed and poor) seldom provide sustained care in the hands of a single clinician throughout treatment. Facilities (e.g., hospital, clinic, and rehabilitation) may or may not be administratively linked, but the patient is confronted with a clinician who is a stranger each time there is an abrupt change in clinical status. Furthermore, therapy is compartmentalized as though no need existed for a primary caretaker to be fully and continuously informed across the domains of data seen as central to one therapy or another.

THE DEVELOPMENTAL INTERACTIVE MEDICAL MODEL REQUIRES A BROAD APPROACH

Schizophrenic illness strikes at the foundations of human functioning. The number of noteworthy problems associated with this type of psychopathology are legion. Similarly, a wide range of defense mechanisms, coping strategies, and personal strengths are relevant to overcoming or adapting to illness. These sweeping implications of schizophrenia for human functioning provide numerous pitfalls for investigator and clinician, but the very complexity of this disorder also creates a unique and fascinating challenge. The range of inquiry is broad, the task is often ambiguous, and the skills, knowledge, and synthesizing abilities required of the student of schizophrenia are demanding. Single modality treatment is inadequate, and the days when the clinician could develop skills and knowledge within one theoretical framework and then apply these techniques to all schizophrenic patients are numbered.

TIME AND TIMING ARE CRUCIAL THROUGHOUT ALL PHASES OF ILLNESS

Time is a dimension critical to understanding schizophrenia. The interactive developmental model of schizophrenia emphasizes temporal relationships among various domains of functioning. Similarly, treatment considerations shift over time, depending on phase of illness and changing circumstances. A patient who decompensates under stress may require procedures which decrease stress when he is on the verge of decompensation, but during another phase of illness, if severe withdrawal and social isolation are prominent, the same stress-reducing procedures may cause a further deterioration in social functioning. We know of no treatment to be applied without change during long periods of an individual's life. The phase of illness, the circumstances in which the patient lives, and the status of the patient's personal coping strategies are not static.

THE CLINICIAN HAS A RESPONSIBILITY TO ACT IN THE FACE OF UNCERTAINTY AND IN THE ABSENCE OF SCIENTIFICALLY VALIDATED INFORMATION

The investigator's task is the acquisition of new knowledge. This differs from the role of the clinician, who must make decisions and take actions with incomplete understanding and imprecise knowledge. This is especially vexing in planning treatment. The extremes are clear. When a therapeutic strategy is proven ineffective, it should be dropped. When a treatment is shown to be efficacious, the clinician will have the responsibility of determining in which patients during which phase of illness the benefits outweigh the risks. However, the efficacy of many therapeutic approaches is neither proven nor disproven. Some argue that treatments only be used after "scientific evidence" supports their efficacy. "Scientific proof" has come to mean double-blind controlled studies, but this standard has been met by only a small fraction of treatments used throughout medicine. The clinician cannot escape the responsibility for sorting through potential therapies and applying them as appropriately as possible with the individual patient.

Two general guidelines enable one to maneuver sensibly through this morass. First, a treatment which conforms to common clinical sense, which can be used to the gratification of patient and/or clinician, and which does not impose undue hazard, should be used when the clinician thinks it is indicated until definitive evidence for lack of efficacy is provided. For example, with insufficient data to reach a conclusion as to whether individual psychotherapy enhances object relations function in the schizophrenic patient, the clinician is wise to consider psychotherapy as a potentially beneficial interpersonal strategy. This is a sensible conclusion based on an understandable body of observation and theory and is not unduly hazardous. Second, treatments without a straightforward clinical rationale, which pose inordinate risk, and which fail to be intuitively valued by clinician and/or patient should be held in abeyance until clinical investigators have established efficacy. For example, hemodialysis may or may not be therapeutic in some schizophrenic patients, but hardships associated with the treatment are considerable, a convincing clinical rationale is missing, and the risks are significant. These considerations justify withholding hemodialysis as a treatment for a schizophrenic patient until efficacy has been demonstrated.

Thus, we do not agree with some workers in the field who advocate the general withholding of therapeutic procedures until their efficacy is established. Rather, we would urge the clinician to apply a broad range of potentially efficacious strategies in the attempt to treat the schizophrenic patient, avoiding unproven treatments with significant risk until evidence for efficacy is presented.

THE BASIC PRINCIPLES OF TREATMENT ARE APPLICABLE FOR ALL SCHIZOPHRENIC PATIENTS

While patients with schizophrenia can have the broadest possible range of outcome functioning, many schizophrenic patients ae unemployed, are handicapped in advocating on their own behalf, and have personal and social support systems that are severely compromised. All too often, treatment is not based on sound principles but rather is limited to the particular therapeutic philosophies of the host institutions, the individual clinicians, or the patient's capacity to pay.

We believe that the fundamental principles on which evaluation and treatment of schizophrenic patients are based are applicable to all patients and are not dependent upon a particular therapeutic philosophy or upon the social and economic support systems available to the patient. If clinical care principles were actually respected, the care of schizophrenic individuals would be radically altered from that which exists today. We are impatient with those who say that circumstances preclude adherence to these principles, although we recognize that the pressures of time, space, and clinical urgency often make it difficult. But much more is possible within the confines of present resources, when the clinical perspective, rather than expediency, shapes therapeutic attitude and administrative policy. The greatest pressure to change should be directed at those health professionals, administrators, and political institutions that have been negligent in failing to advocate sound clinical principles as the only *acceptable* standard for humane care of schizophrenic patients. The person with schizophrenia remains a genuinely disenfranchised member of society.

Index